Majorana Magic Warburg Extrapolation

Deceptive Selective Reporting

MICROSOFT COMPANY NON-

TRUE MAJORANA MAGIC

AF675942

DR. THOMAS SEYFRIED NOBEL PRIZE

CANCER RESOLUTION AND REMISSION

Charles R Giardina

A study: Involving two breakthroughs baffling scientists for almost a hundred years. Based on a common sense approach involving unhinged media reporting and their total exclusion of the proven facts. Both discoveries worthy of Nobel Prizes, when verified using the scientific method.

The first quantum leap, extrapolates the Warburg hypothesis, and news media were silent! Specifically, the discovery of the necessary and sufficient energy sources to sustain cancer. Here, Dr. Thomas Seyfried proved that the amino acid glutamine, along with glucose is all that is needed for cancer growth. By taking the fuel away would kill tumor cells. Fatty acids and ketones can be utilized by normal cells, but not by cancerous cells. He developed a non toxic cancer management technique. It involves very low carbohydrate intake, exercise and periodic low dosages of glutamine inhibiting substances. Dr. Seyfried showed the use of anti parasitic drugs are very successful in preventing cancer metastases, and minimizing their effects.. His treatment results in a much higher quality of living and overall extended life expectancy as compared to the current standard of care. However, again a lack of media presence for this great discovery.

The second quantum leap was a false alarm. It was an exaggerated claim for the existence, observation and control of the subatomic particle the Majorana fermion at a zero energy state. For nearly a century scientists have tried in vein to detect a Majorana particle. This year, worldwide newspapers, magazines, as well as radio and television channels went wild boasting of Microsoft's findings. A beautiful designed, but misleading configuration. It's functioning in a quantum computer needs to be housed in a zero degree vacuum configuration the size of a car. Additionally, numerous other controlling and observing structures are necessary but are external to this processor. However, a ridiculously large amount of attention was provided for a specious result.

Herein, the Chapters and Appendices within this document describe:

- Deserving a Nobel Prize
- Energy is Everything
- Quantum Antiparticles
- Braiding Groups
- Majorana Zero Modes

A tragedy in the history of medicine is: Almost all cancer therapies are based on genetics, toxic poisons, radiation or surgical mutilations. Cancer therapeutics have been conducted over and over with the same methods and always expecting different results. This is a sign of stupidity as well as arrogant ignorance based on medical myths. The present cancer managing system is severely broken. There has to be a paradigm shift. A large part of the current document is grounded on the scientific, objective fact based discoveries by the distinguished scientist Dr. Seyfried. (Seyfried, et al, 2022). His foundational discovery, there is one cancer. Glucose and glutamine synergistically work together to feed cancer. Tumors cannot survive on ketones or fatty acids, they do not need oxygen to respire and always ferment in the creation of energy. Cancerous tissues might utilize oxygen but only to produce Reactive Oxygen Species, ROS which causes mutations within the DNA. Cancer cells have a chronic destruction of OXPHOS and not an acute destruction. When acute disruption occurs the cell dies. Mitochondria always control the state of cells within the human body.

Charles R Giardina

Copyright © 2025 Charles R Giardina. All rights reserved for data mining, text, A.I. and quantum technologies and similar training.

CONTENTS

PREFACE

Two scientific discoveries are described within this document. Both involve energy conversion and production and both, if true are worthy of a Nobel Prize. In both cases, theoretical foundations were established almost a century ago.

The first discovery, 100% scientifically sound, verified, and openly published, is the theory of One Cancer. Cancer is not a somatic theory. It is a metabolic disease. Specifically, cancer is due to the dysfunction of the mitochondria fermenting to create energy. This theory is pioneered by Dr. Thomas Seyfried who extrapolated the works of Nobel Prize winner Dr. Otto Warburg. The latter showed cancer thrives on glucose. Dr. Seyfried proved that the only other substance needed for cancer survival is glutamine. Together these fuels ferment creating lactic and succinic acids. For years, world wide attention did not exist for either of these discoveries. Mainstream news media avoid reporting this amazing research even though Dr. Seyfried provides a non toxic approach to cancer management and cancer remission.

The second revelation, an exaggerated claim for the existence, observation and control of the subatomic particle the Majorana fermion at a zero energy state. For almost 100 years scientists have tried in vein to detect a Majorana particle. Early in 2025, worldwide newspapers, magazines, as well as radio and television channels went wild boasting of Microsoft's findings. Even politicians got involved. The Majorana 1 processor was held up on the floor of the US Senate. A beautiful designed, but misleading configuration. It's functioning in a quantum computer need be housed in a zero degree vacuum configuration the size of a car. Additionally, numerous other controlling and observing structures are necessary but are external to this processor.

The Majorana 1 processor is an indium arsenic aluminum topological superconducting device housing eight qubits. The objective, is to extend topological substances enabling a large number of qubits. Ultimately having quantum computers capable of breaking current security codes. This is the principal application of quantum computing.

1) THE NOBEL PRIZE

1.1) Deserving a Nobel Prize, Who Should Be a Receiver?

Who Should receive a Nobel Prize: A person whose discovery involves the resolution to the most important problem understood by everyone. Surely, Dr. Thomas Seyfried has to be a recipient. He demonstrated the true theory of a single cancer, leading to remission of this disease. His thesis is that cancer is a metabolic dysfunction of the mitochondria caused by fermentation rather than respiration. He extrapolated the famous results of Warburg. Cancer is not a Somatic disease. (Seyfried, and Shelton, 2010). Gene defects are a secondary result, with all gene deficiencies just predispose development of cancer. Gene mutations always have a probability less than one for cancer development. Gene theory for the cause of cancer is ideological dogma. The truth is that cancer cells can only survive on both glucose and the amino acid glutamine. They cannot survive on ketones and fatty acids. His solution for cancer remission is minimization of the use of glucose and employ drugs to inhibit glutamine pathways. (Lee, et al, 2024). Diet, exercise and lifestyle play a major factor in cancer formation. Minimizing glucose intake and modifying glutamine pathways provides a non toxic treatment for cancer.

Dr. Seyfried extended and generalized the famous Warburg hypothesis. (Seyfried, et al, 2025). This timely crucial result is not widely publicized even though Dr. Seyfried has published over a hundred and fifty refereed technical papers on this subject. In general, oncologists, cancer researchers are not familiar or ignore Dr. Seyfried's discovery. The same goes for politicians, as well as the media.

There is an organized systematic failure of cancer researchers, politicians as well as journalists and the media in acknowledging Dr. Thomas Seyfried's discovery. He provides a non toxic, and non evasive procedure for cancer management. Dr. Seyfried proved that there is one cancer and it is a metabolical dysfunction of the oxidation process within the mitochondrial. His hypothesis is that the necessary and sufficient fuels for cancer survival are glucose and the amino acid glutamine. Discontinuance of both of these substances would kill the cancer as well as the human being. The strategy to be used is first start a drastic reduction in glucose intake, and second modify the paths of glutamine absorption. A consequence, is reduction in tumor size and inhibition of metastasis. Numerous experiments substantiated these assumptions. Over a hundred and fifty peer reviewed scientific papers have been published, all in open access documenting and validating these claims.

At a minimum, damage is done to scientific discovery by not acknowledging Dr. Seyfried's extension and generalization of the claims of Nobel prize winner Dr. Otto Warburg. At an average, there are 70 deaths an hour of U.S. citizens due to cancer, and the rate is increasing. Change of diet and life style along with exercise is the essence for the toxic free cancer remission process. The solution indicated by Dr. Seyfried seems too simple, but it must be universally heard, lives are at stake!

For a couple of years doubts about the somatic theory of gene mutations being a direct cause of cancer has been mentioned, (Monti, et al, 2022). Finally, Dr. Seyfried discovered the cause, dysfunction of the mitochondria to perform respiration. Moreover, he found the necessary and sufficient substances for cancer survival, glucose and glutamine.

1.2) Deserving a Nobel Prize, Who Should Not Be a Receiver?

Who should Not Receive a Nobel Prize: It is Microsoft for providing a false and inflated discovery of a problem understood by a very, very few. It is the experimental verification for the existence of the Majorana fermion at a zero energy state. This particle differs greatly from the more usual Dirac fermions described in Appendix 1. For almost 100 years scientists have tried in vein to detect Majorana fermions. These particles are theoretically proposed to exist by Dr. Ettore Majorana, and are defined in Section 5.1. It was reported that Dr. Majorana went missing at sea in

1937. Some historians claimed that he discovered the subatomic particle the neutron. This claim was made prior to Sir James Chadwick's announcing the existence of this particle in 1932. (Recami, 2017). Neutron bombarding is crucial in the nuclear fission reaction central in the formation of atomic bombs. Being a student of Dr. Enrico Fermi might have given Dr. Majorana insight into harms due to the fission process. Fears of the use of this process for the creation of bombs, might have lead to his disappearance. (Amaldi, 1984).

Even though Microsoft receives a tremendous amount of undeserved press, they provide very deceitful results broadcasted throughout the world. The public often believes what is reported. However, even scientific editors and reviewers of several of their documents provide warnings that their discoveries have not been verified. Microsoft implied that the Majorana qubits have been observed and controlled. This qubit is fundamental for the workings of their Majorana One Processor reported by Microsoft in Nature. Microsoft claims quantum-computing breakthrough—but physicists are skeptical, (Castelvecchi, 2025). However, the article in Nature suggests the possibility of measurement techniques provided in the paper are useful in future quantum Majorana based computers. In, (Jainendra, 2025), it was asked if Microsoft's quantum 'breakthrough' revolutionize computing?

Numerous other technical papers exist blasting untruths provided by Microsoft. Additionally, corrected studies rekindle debates over Microsofts's quantum computing research. References can be found in (Mann, 2025). Additionally, in (Garisto, 2025), controversial quantum-computing paper gets hefty correction-but concerns linger. Physicists are mostly unconvinced by Microsoft's new topological chip. (Connover, 2025), Microsoft quantum computing 'breakthrough' faces fresh challenge, (Garisto, 2025). Even some top physicists called Microsoft's claims about observing and controlling Majorana fermions a fraud. Specifically, University of Pittsburg professor Dr. Sergey Frolov claims Microsoft's work here is an "essentially a fraudulent project", (Fox, 2025).

1.3) Facts Involving The Nobel Prize

For almost all scientific disciplines, any hypothesis about the existence of a substance or the workings of a process must be verified by experimentation. Measurements have to be taken and relevant data must be preserved, analyzed and reviewed. Additionally, explorations must lead to observations which are repeatable and validated for truth. Numerous measurements must be conducted and the results have to be replicated under specified conditions. This is called the scientific method. The only field of study where experimentation is not at all needed is in the area of the Queen of Science - Mathematics. Here, a formal factual structure exists. Rigorous proofs are the only means of establishing the correctness of mathematical assumptions. An amazing fact is that there is no Nobel Prize awarded in the field of mathematics. However, mathematicians can receive the Nobel Prize while working in other scientific areas.

In 1965, the explanation for why there is no Nobel Prizes awarded in the field of mathematics was provided to me while at Carnegie Tech. Dr. Zeev Nehari, famous for the Nehari Manifold, related the reason suggested to him by his thesis adviser, Dr. Michael Fekete. While lecturing on the Mittag-Leffler expansion for meromorphic functions, Professor Nehari, indicated that Gosta Mittag-Leffler had an affair with a mistress of Alfred Nobel. The latter person was a famous Swedish chemist. He had an assumed dislike of Mittag-Leffler, while being a friend with King Oscar of Sweden. Five years after Nobel's death, the first Nobel Prize was awarded.

Six areas for Nobel Prizes can be awarded yearly since 1901. These awards are in the categories of: Physics; Chemistry; Physiology and Medicine; Economics; Literature; Peace. (The Nobel Prize Internet Archive, 1996). A listing of Nobel Prize winners up to 2024 can be found in (All Nobel Prizes, 2024).

2) ENERGY IS EVERYTHING

2.1) Energy Conversion in Physiology

Energy is a central concept in all areas of physical as well as biological sciences. This is particularly true in physiology. Here, within the human body potential energy, food, water, H_2O and Oxygen, O are utilized in creating kinetic energy. Thousands of trillions of mitochondria are organelles existing within the body. These structures are mainly focused on energy production. They produce kinetic energy in units of ATP, Adenosine TriphosPhate. Without ATP cells could die. This is true when ATP reduction is sudden, however, when energy production is slowly degrading, chronic diseases such as cancer can result. Under normal conditions, humans breath in oxygen to produce ATP and simultaneously expire H_2O, and CO_2. The process is called respiration, H_2O, is Water and CO_2 is Carbon Dioxide. An in-depth explanation of the normal respiration process can be found in Mysteries of the Mitochondria. (Giardina, 2025). Krebs Cycle, electronic transport chain, and chemiosmosis are detailed in this reference.

In the 1930s, Dr. Otto Warburg showed the Warburg hypothesis, cancer cells can make ATP, that is kinetic energy without the use of oxygen. (Apple, 2021). This is called the fermentation process. Cancer thrives on glucose to produce bodily energy within the mitochondria by fermentation sources. In the fermentation process lactic acid is respired. Even though Dr. Warburg was a Nobel Prize winner, his theory that glucose tremendously increases tumor growth, is ignored. Patients with cancer simultaneously are injected with chemo toxic substances and eat or drink sugar products. This is a criminal offense, and will be verified and validated in due time. The arrogant ignorance of oncologists and others are possibly linked to prejudice reasons.

Recently, Dr.Thomas Seyfried extended and generalized the Warburg hypothesis. He showed the necessary and sufficient fuels to sustain cancer are glucose and the amino acid glutamine. Acid byproducts also occur as glutamine fuels cancer cells, in this case it is succinic acid. Dr. Seyfried identified two major pathways for the fermentation process to exist. One which utilizes glucose outside the mitochondria. The other uses glutamine to create ATP within the mitochondria. This occurs with or without the use of oxygen. When oxygen is employed it creates Reactive Oxygen Species, ROS and this substance mutates the nucleus DNA. Metabolic explanation of Dr. Seyfried's discovery of the fermentation process in cancer is described in Theranostics, (Giardina, 2025). In this non normal process ATP is created by fermentation methods both within and outside of the mitochondria.

Dr. Seyfried's solution for cancer management is simple. It is to change the potential energy needed in sustaining cancer. Starve cancerous cells and halt fermentation by reducing carbohydrates and periodic blocking of the glutamine pathways. The latter technique is called the Press-Pulse strategy. Normal cells can survive on fatty acids and ketones, however, cancerous cells cannot utilize these fuels. Over a hundred fifty highly regarded peered reviewed scientific technical papers have been published on this subject by Dr Seyfried. Ingenious experiments were conducted to illustrate and verify his hypothesis. These were repeated numerous times to make adjustments and validating his findings. All publications exist in open access.

Cancer is a metabolic mitochondria dysfunction involving fermentation and not a genetic disease. This was proved using nucleus and mitochondrial translocations within cancerous and non cancerous cells. Previously mentioned, cancer cells might utilize oxygen but it creates, ROS causing mutations within the nucleus DNA. DNA mutations are an effect, and not a cause for cancer. Moreover, Dr. Seyfried developed an in depth cancer management procedure that emphasizes a high quality of life, and non toxic treatment methods. The primary step to be employed under any suspicion of cancer, is for the subject to progress into a state of ketosis. A recommended manner to attain this state is to have a keto to glucose ratio of less than two. While sustaining this ratio, specific drugs which inhibit glutamine pathways are administered in a personalized manner. Precise dosage, duration and frequency are prescribed most often leading to cancer remission and tumor reduction. This is the Press-Pulse method, previously mentioned. Among the drugs administered are repositioned anti-parasitic drugs. High positive correlation exists between the use of these drugs and the tumor reduction process.

2.2) Energy Metabolism in Cancer Metastasis

Cancer metastasis is the spreading of cancer usually from a single site to various other organs and tissues. Over ninety percent of cancer related deaths are due to metastasis. (Li, et al, 2025). An increase in energy is required during cancer metastasis. (Weber, 2016). Dr. Seyfried spent ten years ultimately discovering that macrophages are responsible for the spreading of cancer. Usually, macrophages act as immune cells. Macrophages are the only cells which can move in and out of tissues. They exist in all cells and some white blood cells also form macrophages. Macrophages fuse with cancerous cells spreading cancerous tumors to various parts of the body. Glutamine is the principal fuel for energizing macrophages. Metastasis can be halted with the obstruction of glutamine pathways. (Shelton, et al, 2010).

2.3) Energy Considerations in Majorana Magic

In short, the quest for discovering Majorana particles has greatly shifted. It went from the search for neutrinos to the search for fabricating materials producing particles which equal its antiparticle. From a practical point of view, it was noticed that these materials necessarily needed zero energy to produce these quantities.

Almost all experimental methods utilized in observing Majorana fermions involve controlled environments involving zero energy states. This is particularly true in condensed matter physics where superconductance enables potentially reliable detection of properties of Majorana fermions. Additionally, Majorana Magic can be explained in theory when non-Abelian anyons are localized in zero energy states. The configuration is termed the Majorana Zero Mode, MZM. Actually MZM are held at an energy very near zero. In this mode Majorana particles are usually separated at the ends of a one dimensional superconductor, or on boundaries of a two dimensional surface. Additionally MZMs are also classified as non-charged quasiparticles equaling its antiparticle. They exist within a topological superconductor. Quasiparticles are described in Section 3.2, and antiparticles in Section 3.1.

A superconductor consists of materials which conduct electricity with zero resistance. They have the well known property of the particle hole symmetry. This means that the fermionic creation operation of the energy equals the fermionic annihilation operation on the negative energy. Using this property of superconductors leads to a path for finding the Majorana fermion. That is:

$$\gamma^{\dagger}(0) = \gamma(0).$$

The equation shows that at zero energy, creation and annihilation are equal, implying a particle equals its antiparticle. Topology involves invariance under continuous deformation of substances. Never tearing or ripping.

It is proposed, by utilizing extreme positions within superconductors, Majorana particles can be employed as highly efficient fault tolerant qubits. Ultimately, within a quantum computer. Separation of Majorana particles improves coherence, allowing a longer time period for the control and observation of qubits. The overall goal is minimizing the loss of quantum information. The need for additional error correction is also lessened due to the particles locations at wire or boundary extremities.

•

The MZM are charge neutral fermionic particles which are zero energy solutions of the Bogolubov de Gennes, BdG equation. The solution usually arises as a topological superconducting state. An important reference is (Chenn and Sigal, 2019). Also, of importance, are Broken Cooper pairs. These are called Bogoliubov quasiparticles. (Giardina, 2024). In superconducting material holes combine with Cooper pairs, and form electrons. (Frolov, 2012).

3) QUANTUM PARTICLES AND QUASIPARTICLES

3.1) Quantum Particles, and Antiparticles

The following decreasing subset sequence follow:

In Physiology; the body contains organs which are comprised of tissues, and they contain cells. Most cells contain, mitochondria and nuclei.

In the standard model of Particle Physics; matter contains molecules and these contain atoms, isotopes and ions. All atoms contain protons and electrons and all but Hydrogen, H also contain neutrons. Isotopes of an atom have the same number of protons as the atom itself. They possess more or less or equal number of neutrons than protons. An ion has more or less electrons than does the specific atom.

Protons and neutrons and electrons are sub-atomic particles. Electrons are classified as elementary particles. Elementary particles have intrinsic properties including mass, electric charge, color charge and spin. Two additional elementary particles are noted next. These involve the most important components of matter. Specifically, the up and down quarks. These are subatomic particles a are located within, and comprise neutrons and protons. The up quark has a positive 2/3 a charge of an electron and a mass of 2 MeV. (Pasayten.org, 2025). While a down quark has a negative charge 1/3 that of an electron and a mass of 5 MeV.

A proton is comprised of two up quarks and a single down quark. Therefore, it has a positive charge equivalent to an electron in absolute value. A neutron is made up of two down quarks and a single up quark. This subatomic particle is charge neutral. In numerous references the mass of neutrons and protons are said to be the same. Additionally, the mass of an electron is assumed to be zero. The actual atomic masses are described relative to the mass of a single neutron, (LibreTexts, 2019):

Neutron mass =1

Proton mass = .9986 · mass of a Neutron

Electron mass = .00054 · mass of a Neutron

Energy is Everything! Two solutions for energy exists for quadratic equations. These involve positive energies and negative energy. Specifically, for mass m and momentum p the energy squared involves the speed of light c:

$$E^2 = p^2c^2 + m^2c^4$$

The solution of this equation involves two branches:

$$E = +/-(p^2c^2 + m^2c^4)^{1/2}$$

The antiparticles are associated with negative energy solutions. (LibreTexts, 2025). Antiparticles or formally, antimatter are names used in referring to physical substances having mostly the same features as the particle itself but often of opposite charge. Sometimes charge need not be a property of antiparticles. For Bosons antiparticles are not unusual, a photon is its own antiparticle. Antiparticles have differing names in diverse areas of physics. A prime example is in semiconducting devices where an antiparticle for an electron is called a hole. This matter is identical to an electron except that the charge is the same as an electron, but it is positive. When an electron leaves the valence band and jumps to the conduction band, a hole is formed. These two particles are attracted by the Coulomb force and form an exciton. The process is named electrical excitation. (Lee, 2025). In the area of nuclear radiation beta particles are often emitted in nuclear fission process. Typically they too are electrons, denoted by β = e. However, often beta particles with all the characteristics of an electron are emitted but they are of positive charge, denoted by β^+. These antiparticles in most areas of physics are called positrons.

Antiparticles are crucial in nuclear imaging as well, namely for Positron Emission Tomography, PET. When particles and antiparticles combine different names are also provided for the combined substances. In PET machines, positrons are formed due to radio active substances injected into patients. As fast as positrons are formed they collide with electrons and form positroniums.

Subsequently, this combined substance of little mass is almost instantly annihilated, and converted into two 511keV of gamma ray energies. These rays are observed by PET cameras and are used in image creation. See (Giardina, 2025) for descriptions of nuclear and radioactive imaging. An excellent mathematical description of positroniums is provided in (Kiessaling, 2018).

In 1937 Dr. Ettore Majorana proposed the existence of a particle which is its own antiparticle. He claimed that the neutrino might be such a particle. But this has never been established. These particles have no charge and essentially no mass. Actually, they have a millionth mass of an electron. However a neutrino has helicity, that is a counter clockwise spin whereas an antineutrino has a clockwise spin. Exploiting the helicity aspect of neutrinos are being used to confirm Majorana's conjecture. However, due to the negligible mass of a neutrinos, other methods are used in hopes of observing a Majorana particle. See the next section, where the search for quasiparticles took over. In any case, both neutrinos or antineutrinos occur from the decay of isotopes from specific atoms. As an instance of neutrino discharge is provided below.

Example 3.1)

In 12.9 minutes after its creation a nitrogen isotope $^{13}_{7}$N, decays by half into a carbon isotope $^{13}_{6}$C. Here, the atomic mass of both N and C is 13, but the atomic number of C is one less than N. Additionally, the emission of a positive beta particle β^+, is illustrated below along with a neutrino,

$$^{13}_{7}\text{N} \text{ ---> } ^{13}_{6}\text{C} + \beta^+ + \text{neutrino.}$$

As previously mentioned β^+ doesn't travel far and hits an electron, e, creating a positronium. Subsequently, it gets annihilated. Two photons are emitted, typically in this case, 180 degrees apart. It is these two gamma rays that the gamma cameras within PET, must capture.#

3.2) Quasiparticles

Before quasiparticles are described it is important to mention that these structures are sometimes not well defined. Objects have features or attributes and features have values. Frequently, quasiparticles are defined by values tagged to various features. However, these values are often not necessary and sufficient to uniquely identify the structure. Values are almost always numerical, they could be binary. In this case, *Yes* signifieds a one, or *No* denotes a zero. For instance, in condensed matter physics the Majorana particle is classified as a quasiparticle. Properties of quasiparticles are neutral in charge, they do not annihilate each other, they are their own antiparticle. Additionally, they come in separate parts, and when paired form a quantum state. Finally, when two such particles are juxtaposed actually transposed, the quantum state changes in a predictable but non commutative manner.

The search for Majorana particles are more currently linked to the search for anyons. These are not bosons nor fermions. The exist in dimension two or less. The reason for associating anyons with Majorana particles is that both exhibit non Abelian statistics. In particular, the MZM is classified as a non Abelian anyon equaling its antiparticle. It exists at zero energy. This substance is often localized within superconductors at topological defects such as edges or vortices. Vortices are illustrated in Figure 3.1, and are described in Section 3.5. The original and most fundamental research paper proposing the existence of anyons is mentioned next.

In 1977 it was proposed, (Leinaas and Myrheim, 1977) that the traditional methods for classifying bosons or fermions is not applicable to a restricted two dimensional particle movement. This was the first hint on the existence of anyons. Prior to 2020 there were only two types of particles known to exist, Bosons and Fermions. These particles form the foundation of the two distinct Fock spaces, and are described in Appendix 1. Details of the ladder operators, creation and annihilation form the algebraic foundation for Fock space. Examples of Fermions include particles within most atoms such as protons, neutrons as well as electrons. Often these types of particles repel each other. Quarks are also Fermions, and these subatomic particles make up protons and neutrons.

Quarks are held in position within both protons and neutrons using a glue type or force binding substance called gluons. These are massless particles and are a type of boson. Just like photons which are also Bosons, gluons bunch together. It is also true the the Hydrogen atom, ${}_{1}^{1}H$ having a single proton and a single electron both being fermions is itself a boson. The notation, ${}_{1}^{1}H$, implies that the lower one is the number of protons in the atom. The upper one is the sum of protons plus neutrons, thus, there are no neutrons in Hydrogen.

Based on Bose Einstein statistics or characteristics within Bosonian Fock space, the wave form identity is provided. Here, the 180 degree rotation of two Bosons, x_1, x_2 within a plane have wave functions $\psi(x_1, x_2) = \psi(x_2, x_1)$. More generally, for the transposition, $\psi(x_1, x_2, \ldots x_i, \ldots x_j, \ldots x_k) = \psi(x_1, x_2,$

... x_j,,... x_i,... x_k), x_i is not equal to x_j. Accordingly, a 360 degree rotation results in an identity. For Fermions, the 180 degree rotation of two Fermions, x_1, x_2 within a plane have wave functions $\psi(x_1, x_2) = - \psi(x_2, x_1)$. More generally, $\psi(x_1, x_2, ..., x_i,... x_j,...x_k) = -\psi(x_1, x_2, ... x_j,..., x_i,... x_k)$. This result is consistent with the Fermi-Dirac statistics. Again, as with Bosons a full rotation of 360 degrees results in the original wave function. In short, the transposition exchange statistics for a Boson involves a phase of $e^{i0} = 1$, and for a Fermion it is $e^{i\pi} = -1$.

3.3) Quantum Particles With Intermediate Exchange Statistics

Anyons have intermediate exchange statistics between Bosons and Fermions. Superconducting quantum computers use transistor wires to hold quantum information. Typical superconducting qubits work electrons pair up into Cooper pairs which become Bosons. Since they are Bosons they bind together, and the whole wire becomes a quantum substance. The result is a Boson condensation type of quantum computing. The whole wire acts as a quantum state. Trapped ions are Fermionic. Press announcement by Microsoft, Anyonic quantum computing. 180 degree shift followed by another 180 degree rotation counterclockwise for Bosons they return to original state. With a braid Boson is identity for switching two particles but for Fermions switching two particles becomes a twisted braid. Swapping particles which are non Abelian Anyons are more complicated, and produce more complex symmetries.

A most important property of braids is that these structures form a non abelian infinite group. This property can be seen in Section 4.2. However the most elegant method of proof is to show this structure is equivalent to a fundamental group, Artin braid group. A rigorous derivation is provided in StackExchange, (Reid, 2014), An easy to read description of fundamental groups and homotopy groups can be found in (Giardina, 2024). Additionally, an introductory description of fundamental groups is briefly described in Appendix 2 of this document.

Based on (Kitaev, 2001), spin less fermions in one dimension superconductor are used in creating Majorana zero modes. This results in topological qubit non abelian statistics. The definition of Majorana operators are formally specified in Section 5.1. In that section the fermion creation operator, f*, and destruction operators f, are employed where { f, f* } =1. See Appendix A1.3. In semiconductor or superconductor physics f* often denotes an electron, and f denotes a hole. Additionally, Majorana particles are described as a superposition of electrons and holes.

A Majorana particle cannot be found in a semiconductor. It cannot be created by first extracting an electron from a conduction band. Then taking a hole in the valence band. Subsequently, forming a superposition of the two particles. This results in an exciton which is a boson. It has mass two times that of an electron and of zero charge. Also mentioned in Section 3.1. However, the method for forming a Majorana particle in superconductance physics is to form the superposition of a hole with a Cooper pair. In general, there are an arbitrary number of Cooper pairs. This forms a condensate of Cooper pairs.

When a hole is applied an electron is the result. In a superconductor there are two states. One state is when there is an integer number of Cooper pairs, denoting a ground type state. The other state is when there is an extra single electron, or a single hole along with all the Cooper pairs. This denotes an excited state. This practical description is due to Frolov in (Mourik, et al, 2012),

3.4) Quasiparticles Leading to Abelian Anyons

For a long time physicists knew that there were basic particles also called quasiparticles. The most prominent are those comprising atoms. They exist in the three dimensional world. These particles are electrons, protons and neutrons. They all are classified as Fermions, and similar particles usually repel each other. On the other hand, there are other quasiparticles in three dimensional. These basic particles have a tendency to bunch together and are called Bosons. One of the most obvious Boson is a photon of light. Appendix A1, provides a deeper description as well as operators involving Fermions and Bosons. From the late 1970s a third basic particle was guessed to exist. In the mid 1980s, without proof of its existence, this particle was named an Anyon. In the Abelian case, it follows that: the 180 degree rotation of two anyons, x_1, x_2 within a plane have wave functions

$$\psi(x_1, x_2) = e^{i\theta}\, \psi(x_2, x_1).$$

Theta is an angle between zero and pi. Different anyons have different angles. Note that, if $\theta = 0$, a boson appears, and if $\theta = \pi$, a fermion results. For an additional rotation a phase of $e^{i2\theta}$ is a consequence. An outcome is that the particle does not return to its original position.

It wasn't until 2020 that experiments proved the existence of commutative Anyons in two dimensional systems. For almost two decades prior to the proof of the existence of Anyons, researchers proposed numerous applications for this type of basic particle. Since Anyons existence was not verified during this time these applications can be considered to be mathematical exercises. A time based evolution of several events leading up to the discovery of Abelian Anyons involving quasiparticles follows.

· 1924 Bose Einstein Statistics, originally published by Bose in (Bose, 1924). In 1925, Einstein generalized Bose's results involving photons to atoms.

· 1925 Pauli Principle and Fermi Dirac Statistics, an easy to read description of the latter could be found in (Biswas, 2015). The Pauli exclusion principle is basic to quantum mechanics, and was first introduced for electrons. No two electrons with the same spin can occupy the same quantum number. This principle was extended to fermions in 1940, (Helmenstine, 2022).

· 1936 Ettore Majorana Fermions, predicted the existence of particles which are also their antiparticle. As previously mentioned, he hypothesized that neutrino particles are their own antiparticle. It is still not known if the neutrinos are Majorana fermions, or just Dirac fermions. The search for Majorana particles lately began in different directions, namely searching for quasiparticles, (Scienceinfo.net, 2025). This lead to investigations into the existence of anyons.

· Schrieffer, J., published What is a quasiparticle?, in J of Res NBS,1969. In this publication the origin of mass enhancement and other interactions between quasiparticles are described. Their existence in metals is also detailed. These particles when grouped together have quantifiable physical properties. They work in unison as a whole.

· 1977 J. Leinaas and J. Myrheim published, On the theory of identical particles, in Il Nuovo Cimento B, vol. 37, issue 1, pp 1-23. (NASA/ADS, 1977). This paper describes that the traditional methods for classifying bosons or fermions is not applicable to a restricted two dimensional quasiparticle movement. This is one of the most important theoretical results. It lead to the discovery of commutative anyons, and suggestions of non commutative anyons.

· 1981 Griffin and Talbot published, Theory of neutron scattering from thermally excited quasiparticles in superfluid ^{4}He, Griffin, A., and

Talbot, E., APS, 1981. This paper describes a theoretical study of the inelastic neutron scattering of thermally excited quasiparticles.

· 1982 Frank Wilczek coined the word anyon to those quasiparticles described by Leinaas and Myrheim. He also published two papers relating the fractional statistics to these anyon particles.

· 1984 Halperin, B., published Statistics of quasiparticles and the hierarchy of fractional quantized Hall states in Phys Rev. Let, 52, 1984.

In anticipation of the actual creation or observation of anyons or Majorana particles, hundreds of papers were written proposing semiconductor use as well as superconductance. Additionally, new assemblies and new materials were proposed. Anticipation of these quasiparticles also produced several different architectures and memories for quantum computers, as well as additional theory. A sample follows.

· 1988 Frohlich illustrated that partial exchange can be monoidal and non-Abelian statistics can arise due to system degeneracy.

· 1997 Kitaev reported on topological quantum computing with non-Abelian anyons.

· 2008 Fu and Kane proposed the use of topological insulator using a magnetic field with superconductor Majorana bound states on the surface.

· 2014 Car, D., et al, published, Rationally designed single crystalline nanowire networks, in Advanced Materials. Looking forward to the actual creation of Majorona fermions, nanowire assemblies are formed. Indium Antimony, $_{49}$In $_{51}$Sb, nanowires meeting at an optimal angle shows promise for a random access memory structure.

· 2016 Aasen, D., et al Milestones toward Majorana-based quantum computing, Phys Rev 2016. In this document semiconducting wires are interfaced in superconducting islands. It is hoped that the readout of Majorana Zero Modes can be observed, and then manipulated. Utilization of gate control for tunnel barriers as well as Coulomb effects are suggested to enable observations of MZMs.

· 2016 Vijay, S.,and Fu, L., reported in the Phys Rev, Teleportation-based quantum information processing with Majorana Zero Modes, MZMs. A measurement based scheme for performing the braiding operations on MZMs. Superconducting islands are created in hopes of observing the non Abelian statistics involving MZMs.

· 2017 Karzig, et al, published Scalable designs for quasiparticle-poisoning-protected topological quantum computation with Majorana Zero Modes, Phys Rev, 2017. Scalable quantum computers are suggested using four or more MZMs. Existing at the ends of superconducting wire, and assembled into superconducting islands with a large charging energy. Tunable couplings between MZM and quantum dots are proposed.

3.5) Discovery of Abelian Anyons

As previously mentioned, 1977 it was theorized the existence of a particle subsequently named an Anyon. More than forty years later experiments proved the existence of commutative Anyons in two dimensional systems. A sample of the titles of papers launched during this time is given below along with a brief description:

· 2020 Bartolomei, H., et al, published Fractional statistics in Anyon collisions, Science, 2020. This was the first detection of anyon particles. Experimental demonstrations of Abelian fractional statistics were performed using collisions between anyons involving beamsplitters.

· 2020 Castelvecchi, D., reported in Nature, that physicists at Purdue U exhibited more evidence of the existence of anyons. Here, Nakamura, J., et al, published an internal report on this existence. In any case, the Nature article is titled: Welcome anyons! Physicists find best evidence yet for long-sought 2D structure. They illustrated the collective excitations of many electrons in solid devices exhibiting the anyon's effects.

· 2020 Ornes, S., et al, published, “Physicists probe anyons exist, a third type of particle in the universe-physicists give us an early view of a third kingdom of quasiparticles that only arise in two dimensions, Discover, 2020. This second discovery of Anyons employed an experimental setup on an etched chip.

· 2020 Nakamura, J., et al, published, Direct observation of anyonic braiding statistics at the 1/3 fractional quantum Hall state, AeXiv.

The discovery of Abelian Anyons in a two dimensional plane involving GaAs/AlGaAs type structure based on the last reference above. The area of the square region is $1\mu m$ by $1\mu m$. A simplified representation of an experiment having much in common to the reference, is provided in Figure 3.1. Here, a magnetic field is assumed to be applied perpendicular to the two dimensional plane illustrated in this figure. Moreover, a current source exists connecting the left and right boundaries. Accordingly, electrons flow in the vertical direction within the structure illustrated in the diagram. This produces a voltage difference as measured between the top and bottom edges of the structure. When the temperature of the substance is brought down near absolute zero the voltage increases in integer jumps. This is called the quantum Hall effect. More importantly, the figure below shows vortices or circular paths also called cyclone motion. In certain materials vortices are created by laser movements, (Madison, et al, 2000). Additionally they often appear due to imperfections in the lattice structure. In, (Nakamura, et al, 2020), vortices are described as small circular regions within the interior of this square structure. Moreover, the observation was made that they denote anyonic braiding. When the temperature is reduced to near absolute zero along with disturbances, such as intermittent heating then the voltage increases in fractional integer jumps, called the fractional quantum Hall effect. It is believed that anyons group together to create these fractional voltage jumps. The braiding aspect involving anyons is described in Section 4.4.

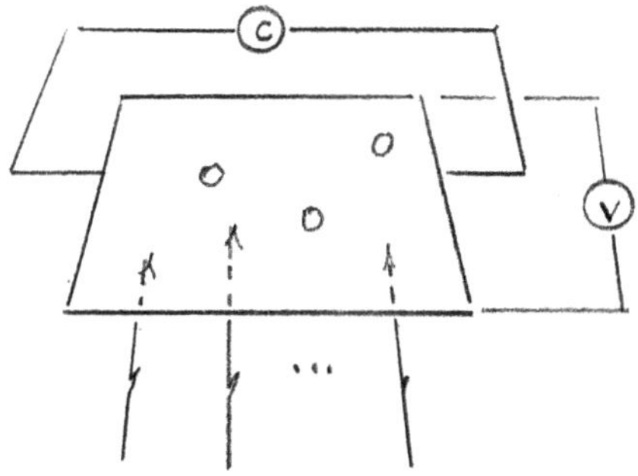

FIGURE 3.1)

In Figure 3.1, the c denotes a current source. It is applied on the left and right boundary. The arrows on the bottom indicate magnetic fields perpendicular to the square substance. The v is the observed voltage induced by this matter. It increases stepwise as the temperature approaches zero. Anyons are indicated by small circles on top of this superconductor.

The existence of non Abelian anyons has not been verified. The non commutativity aspect is claimed to be due to their equivalence with braided sets. Transpositions of anyons are related by unitary matrices.

4) BRAIDING GROUPS

4.1) Configuration Space Braided Sets

The configuration space involves a topological manifold X along with a positive integer k, it is denoted by S(X, k), and is called the k configuration space for X. Also, S(X, k) = { (x_1, x_2, ... , x_k) in X^k, where for i not equal to j, x_i is not equal to x_j }. An intuitive illustrative description of a braid group involving the k configuration space for X begins mainly for points on the real axis or in the x-y plane. In this case, two parallel sets of points separated in the vertical direction one unit apart are used. These points are located in the ordered set (x_1, x_2, ... , x_k). In the more general situation, the space X contains no metric for distance measuring, and no order or no geometry, thus no notion of parallel.

The braided set $B_{k,1}$ consists of k distinct straight lines connecting every point on top to a unique point below. Only neighboring transpositions are allowed or invariant operations, that is identity maps, denoted by I. The identity map means that for every point x_j can only be connected to itself. Or x_j, j = 1, 2,...,k-1 can be connected to a right hand neighboring point x_{j+1}. Or x_j, j = 2,...,k can be connected to a left hand neighboring point x_{j-1}. When such neighbors exist. However, there is one catch, lines which seem to intersect cannot. Crossing lines are illustrated one line on top of another. Lines involving point x_j in a transposition with x_{j+1} are indicated by f_j, when they are above. Therefore, f_j can be perceived as a function mapping x_j into x_{j+1}, it concurrently maps x_{j+1} into x_j, from below. This is symbolized as

$$f_j((x_j, x_{j+1})) = (x_{j+1}, x_j).$$

Lines involving point x_j in a transposition with x_{j+1} are indicated by f_j^{-1}, when they are below. Therefore, f_j^{-1} can be perceived as a function mapping x_j into x_{j+1}, it concurrently maps x_{j+1} into x_j, from above. This is symbolized as

$$f_j^{-1}((x_j, x_{j+1})) = (x_{j+1}, x_j).$$

When the identity map, I is used. Elements within $B_{k,1}$ are called braids or sets of k strands.

Example 4.1)

Suppose that X = R, the real line, and k = 3, then X^3 consists of a set of three points. For instance, the ordered set (x, y, z) is illustrated on top and on the bottom of all images within Figure 4.1. This diagram illustrates the braided set $B_{3,1}$ consisting of five operators. These are illustrated respectively in Figures 4.1, A, B, C, D, and E.

(x, y, z)—->(x, y, z), created by I

(x, y, z)—->(y, x, z) created by f_x

(x, y, z)—->(x, z, y) created by f_y

(x, y, z)—->(y, x, z) created by f_x^{-1}

(x, y, z)—->(x, z, y) created by f_y^{-1}.

In the illustration given below solid lines go over broken lines.#

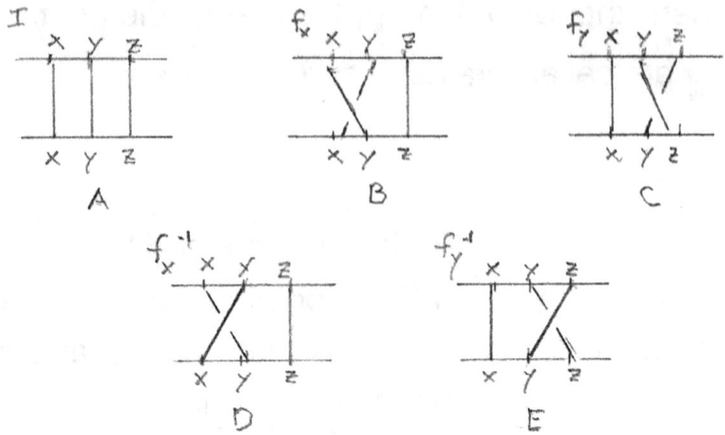

FIGURE 4.1)

The previous example only involved at most a single transposition. When k is greater than 3, disjoint paired couples of points can be involved in multiple transpositions. The next example illustrates this concept by using a multiplication symbol, · . For points m and n involved in disjoint transpositions the symbology is $f_m \cdot f_n = f_n \cdot f_m$. This representation is used when both m and n are involved with lines above. The inverse operator is employed whenever a line is below.

Example 4.2)

Suppose that X = R, the real line, and k = 4, then X^4 consists of a set of four points. For instance the ordered set (x, y, z, u), should be illustrated on top and on the bottom of all images within Figure 4.2. This diagram illustrates the braided set $B_{4,1}$. The following operators are illustrated respectively in Figures 4.2, A, B, C, D, E, F, G, H, I, J, and K.

(x, y, z, u)—->(x, y, z, u), created by I

(x, y, z, u)—->(y, x, z, u) created by f_x

(x, y, z, u)—->(x, z, y, u) created by f_y

(x, y, z, u)—->(x, y, u, z) created by f_z

(x, y, z, u)—->(y, x, u, z) created by $f_x \cdot f_z = f_z \cdot f_x$

(x, y, z, u)—->(y, x, z, u) created by f_x^{-1}

(x, y, z, u)—->(x, z, y, u) created by f_y^{-1}

(x, y, z, u)—->(x, y, u, z) created by f_z^{-1}

(x, y, z, u)—->(y, x, u, z) created by $f_x \cdot f_z^{-1}$

(x, y, z, u)—->(y, x, u, z) created by $f_x^{-1} \cdot f_z$

(x, y, z, u)—->(y, x, u, z) created by $f_x^{-1} \cdot f_z^{-1}$#

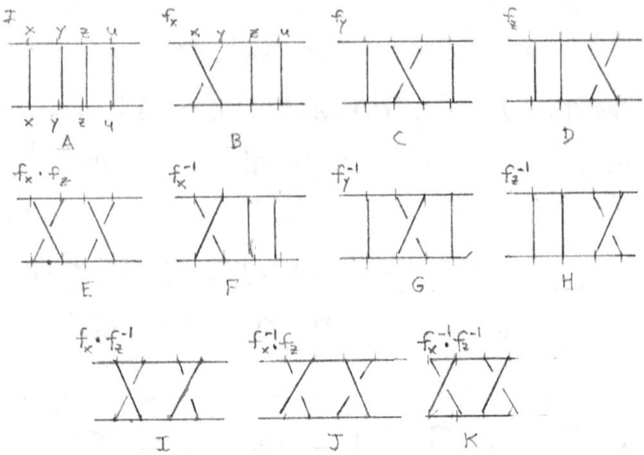

FIGURE 4.2)

4.2) Braided Groups

Elements within braided sets for the same value k should be stacked one underneath the other. By stacking any two elements within the braided set, B $_{k,1}$ produces the elements within set $B_{k,2}$. In the set $B_{k,2}$ braids appear of longer length in this representation. Twice as long. A multiplication type operation, or composition operation is again symbolized using the dot. It is employed involving the creation operator on the upper set · the creation operation in the lower set. However, the operation is this case need not be commutative Several illustrations are provided using $B_{k,2}$ in the Figure 4.3, they are explained in the Example 4.3.

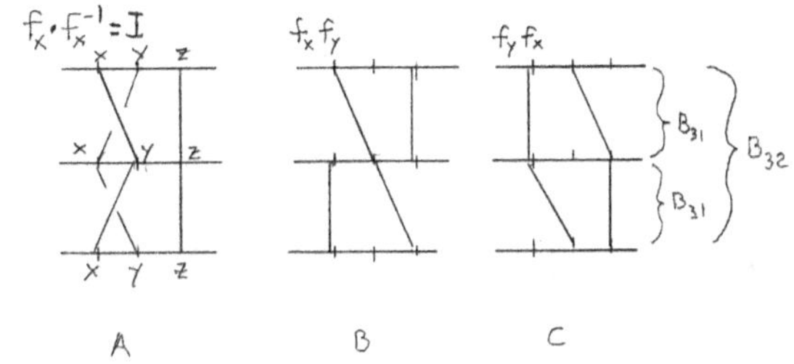

FIGURE 4.3)

Example 4.3)
Refer to Example 4.1) and to Figure 4.3 A, where it is first shown that $f_x \cdot f_x^{-1}$ = I, the identity operation. This follows because from the topmost values, to the bottommost values there are no changes: x—>y—>x, y—>x—>y, and z—>z—>z. In Figure 4.3 B, and C, $f_x \cdot f_y$ is illustrated followed by $f_y \cdot f_x$ respectively. These two elements in $B_{3,2}$ are not equal, showing that the dot operator need not commute. For instance in Figure 4.3 B, x—>y—>z but in Figure 4.3 C, x—>x—>y, the end results differ. #

In a similar manner the set $B_{k,3}$ is found by placing $B_{k,1}$ under $B_{k,2}$. Continuing this process produces a group structure whose elements are braids of longer lengths, and the dot operation is the binary operation for the group. Figure 4.4, illustrates a polygraph depicting the group structure. In general for fixed k there are an infinite collection of braids. Sets of braids within $B_{k,n+1}$ are found by placing braids in $B_{k,1}$ underneath braids located in the set $B_{k,n}$. By this construction existing braids within $B_{k,n}$ are made longer by adhering braids in $B_{k,1}$ underneath. The methodology is called space timeline extension. Intuitively, space refers to horizontal lines indicating the points (x_1, x_2, ... , x_k), used in identifying braid points. A timeline goes downward placing other braids within $B_{k,1}$, under those in $B_{k,n}$, resulting in braids in $B_{k,n+1}$.

The closure operation for a group structure is illustrated in Figure 4.4. In this diagram, the polyadic arrow takes two braids and connects them using the space timeline extension. This represents a binary operator indicated by the dot (·), and the output is also a braid. Additionally, the identity braid I has to be in the group and this is illustrin the diagram as: Identity —-> Set of braids. Finally, the unary operation of inverse is portrayed as an arrow taking a braid f, and providing it's inverse f^{-1}. Note that $(f^{-1})^{-1} = f$.

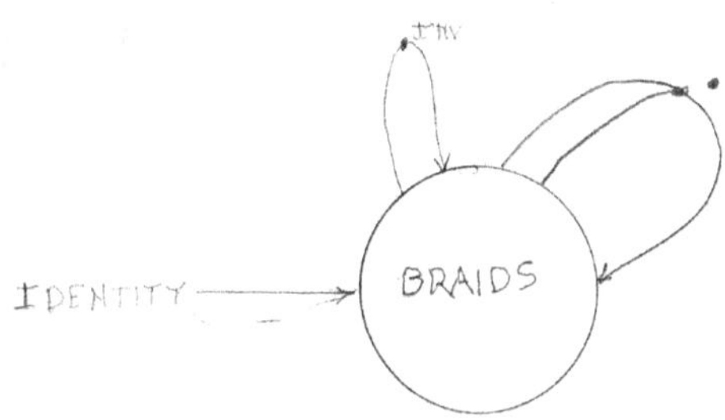

FIGURE 4.4)

The equational constraints for a group structure involving braids, f, g, h and the identity braid I, are:

Associative law, $(f \cdot g) \cdot h = f \cdot (g \cdot h)$

Identity law, $f \cdot I = I \cdot f = f$

Inverse law, $f \cdot f^{-1} = f^{-1} \cdot f = I$.

Example 4.4)

Referring to Example 4.2) where $B_{4,1}$ is utilized three times first by creating ($f_x \cdot f_y$) in $B_{4,2}$, and composing it on the bottom with f_z in $B_{4,1}$. This is illustrated in Figure 4.5 A. Also in Figure 4.5 B, f_x in $B_{4,1}$ is on top and this is followed by ($f_y \cdot f_z$) on the bottom in $B_{4,2}$. The resulting products are equal, illustrating the associative law for a group structure. That is $(f_x \cdot f_y) \cdot f_z = f_x \cdot (f_y \cdot f_z)$.#

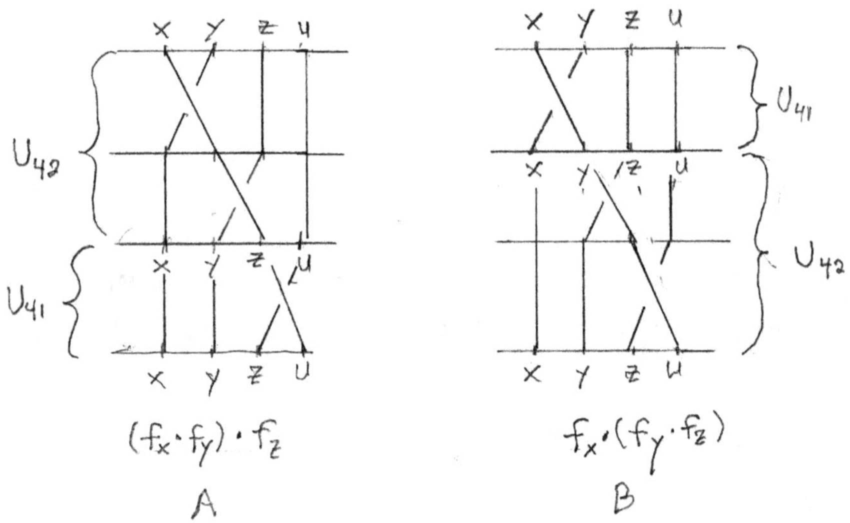

FIGURE 4.5)

For any braid $f_j \cdot f_p \cdot \cdot \cdot f_m \cdot f_q$ in $B_{k,n}$, the inverse operation is $f_q^{-1} \cdot f_m^{-1} \cdot \cdot \cdot f_j^{-1}$. Additionally, similar to the results given in Example 4.2, braids created more than one unit apart do commute. This is in B $_{k,n}$, $f_{x_i} \cdot f_{x_j} = f_{x_j} \cdot f_{x_i}$ whenever $| i - j | > 1$. Moreover, the following mirror image pattern involving three braids within $B_{k,n}$ applies: It is described by a relation, $f_{x_i} \cdot f_{x_j} \cdot f_{x_i} = f_{x_j} \cdot f_{x_i} \cdot f_{x_j}$ whenever, $| i - j | = 1$.

4.3) Equivalent Descriptions of Braided Sets

The use of straight lines connecting points within S(X, k) are usually not employed in describing braids. Instead, curved lines are used. These curved lines are also called strands. Additionally, the length of the braids also does not matter. The strands comprising braids within $B_{k,n}$ can be pulled, pushed, and bent resulting in the morphing of a braid into its equivalent. In general, there is no concept of length and only topological invariants are employed. These invariants involve over or under strand crossovers. Figure 4.6 illustrates different structures representing the same braid as well as a non braided structure.

Example 4.5)
Referring to Figures 4.6 A, and B, these represent the same braid. A simple justification method, but not always applicable can be exhibited by starting on top of each diagram. Then follow the strand for each point in $B_{4,4}$ as if the strand is a highway. Going downward, when en-counting a different highway, record if a bridge is used or a tunnel. A bridge is on top and the tunnel is under. In the first diagram previously mentioned the following holds, and is easy to follow:

Strand x tunnels under y, bridges over z and u to arrive at u
Strand y bridges over x and arrives at x
Strand z tunnels under y and z to arrive at z
Strand u tunnels under z then bridges over y to arrive at y.

These braids are easy to follow when $B_{4,4}$ is partitioned into four copies of $B_{4,1}$. Starting from the top set $B_{4,1}$ the operator f_x^{-1} is applied. For the subsequent sets underneath, going top down, the operators are shown, in order f_y, f_z, and f_y^{-1} respectively. In Figure 4.6 B, starting in configuration (x, y, z, u) and winding up in configuration (u, x, z, y) can be traced, but with more difficulty than in Figure 4.6 A. Also notice that Figure 4.6 C, and D are also equivalent. Notice in these diagrams it is more obvious that the strand z stays invariant. Also, note that Figure 4.6 D, shows that the braids can be wiggly, the only important thing is that there cannot be any knots. Figure 4.6 E, illustrates a non braid structure since there are knots or self loops.#

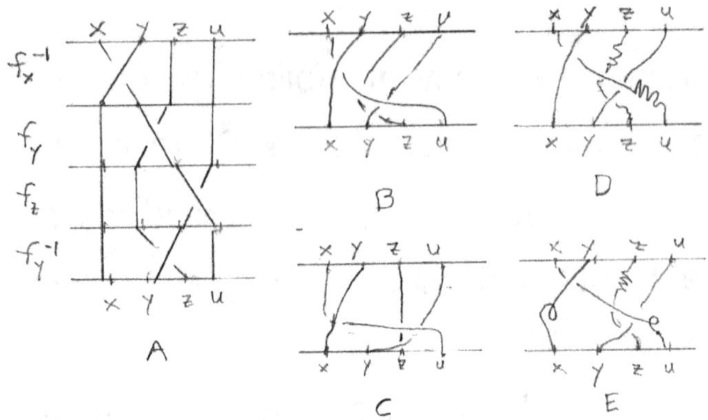

FIGURE 4.6)

In general, showing the equivalence of braids is not simple. The method illustrated in the above example is difficult to apply in general, due to the nonuniform lengths and curvatures of braids. Moreover, there may be equivalence, but the method fails. See Figure 4.3 A.

4.4) Braided Sets of Anyons

Anyons are braided for application of Topological Quantum Computing, TQC. Figure 4.7 illustrates four anyons x, y, z, and u forming braids to approximate actual unitary matrix gates. World lines show the progression of braids. World lines are formed by counter clockwise rotation of anyons within the two dimensional plane. As time increases going downward, world lines are intertwined from movement in the flat world. Sometimes tunneling occurs in the braiding process.

An interesting paper on tunneling involving the time domain braiding of anyons is provided in, (Ruelle, et al, 2024). Abelian anyons have fractional quantized Hall effect, fluctuation of quantum systems. Non-Abelian wave function are governed by unitary usually non commutative transformations creating a new wave function. Topological braiding of unitary matrices are illustrated in Figure 4.7. In these diagrams robust time world lines shows time progressing downward. A configuration space consisting of four anyons (x, y, z, u) is utilized in this diagram.

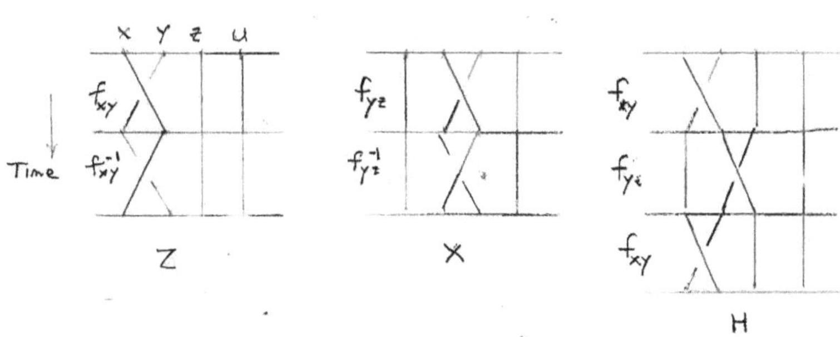

FIGURE 4. 7)

Several actual matrices utilized in quantum computing are, the Pauli X, Pauli Z, and Pauli Y:

$$\begin{vmatrix} 0 & 1 \\ 1 & 0 \end{vmatrix} \qquad \begin{vmatrix} 1 & 0 \\ 0 & -1 \end{vmatrix} \qquad \begin{vmatrix} 0 & -i \\ i & 0 \end{vmatrix}.$$

Additionally, the rotation, phase and 45 degree matrices are respectively, $R_{i\phi}$, S and T

$$\begin{vmatrix} 1 & 0 \\ 0 & e^{i\phi} \end{vmatrix} \qquad \begin{vmatrix} 1 & 0 \\ 0 & i \end{vmatrix} \qquad \begin{vmatrix} 1 & 0 \\ 0 & e^{i\pi/4} \end{vmatrix}.$$

Finally, among the most important matrices is the Hadamard, it is given by $2^{1/2}H =$

$$\begin{vmatrix} 1 & 1 \\ 1 & -1 \end{vmatrix}.$$

Explanation of these matrices can be found in (Giardina, 2024).

Creation of braids to be used in TQC are frequently approximations of unitary matrices and are often performed by by brute force searching methods. (Rouabah, 2008). In this reference an approximation H' to the Hadamard matrix H was found such that the error ϵ = .00657.

For arbitrary unitary target matrix U, and braided approximation W, the formula for error is:

$$\epsilon(W, U) = [2 - tr(WU^*].$$

Where tr is the trace or sum of diagonal element within the product WU*. Here U* is the conjugate transpose of U. In the above reference, thirty levels of braiding was employed in giving,

$$\epsilon(H', H) = .00657.$$

Using the notation Section 4.1 H' represents a braided set within $B_{4,30}$. Also see (Rouabah, et al, 2020).

Global effect matters. New wave functions arise as the twisting of braids involving anyons. on two dimensional planes proceed downward as time increases on world lines.

Topological quantum gates are slightly effected by noise when anyons are braided. Topological gates are a function of the fundamental group, that is the homotopy class of braids are involved., (Alicia, et al, 2011)

5) MAJORANA PARTICLES

5.1) Majorana Zero Modes

The Majorana Zero Mode, MZM is best explained using ideas of Kitaev, (Kitaev, 2001) Kitaev, A., Unpaired Majorana particles in quantum wires, Physics, 2001. The model utilized is called the Kitaev-Majorana chain, and does not prove the existence of Majorana particles. It is a single dimensional semiconducting nanowire used in illustrating quantum topology. Zero temperature is assumed. Figure 5.1 A, denotes chains of Dirac fermions f_1, f_2, ..., f_N, Additionally, chains are given underneath correspondingly consisting of their real parts a_i, and imaginary parts b_i. The fermions are said to be spin-less because they all are assumed to be of the same spin, say upward. Practically, a P wave superconductivity forces all electron spins to occur in the same direction. A more practical description of the Kitaev-Majorona chain is provided by Frolov in (Mourik, et al, 2012). In this referenced paper guidelines are provided for conducting experiments proposing the existence of Majorona particles. They specify the use of a one dimensional wire along with a spin orbit interaction for creating a single directional spin of electrons. Also the use of superconductive materials along with magnetic fields are needed in this construction.

In Figure 5.1 A, each actual Dirac fermion is theoretically composed of two Majorana particles, indeed, $f_j = 1/2(a_j + ib_j)$. The Majorana particles are $a_j = f_j + f_j^{\dagger}$, and $b_j = i(f_j^{\dagger} - f_j)$. When viewed as operators, $f_j^{\dagger}$, is the creation and f_j is the annihilation operator. The Hamiltonian H for the chain model is given below, (Kitaev, 2001). It is given here to describe how two Majorana particles are created a far distance from each other at different ends of the chain.

$$H = \sum_{j=1}^{N-1}[(\Delta f_j^{\dagger} f_{j+1}^{\dagger} + t f_j^{\dagger} f_{j+1}) + (\Delta f_j^{\dagger} f_{j+1}^{\dagger} + t f_j^{\dagger} f_{j+1})^{\dagger}] - u \sum_{j=1}^{N} f_j^{\dagger} f_j.$$

The quantity Δ denotes the pairing term, it specifies the coupling between neighboring creation or annihilation operators. Additionally, t is referred to as the hopping term which describes the kinetic energy involving these operations. The foundation for the Kitaev chain model is the Hubbard model given in (U of Rhode Island, 2011). Finally u is the chemical potential, which indicates the amount of energy changes due to the addition or removal of fermions. Assuming that u = 0 and Δ = t, then the Hamiltonian becomes:

$$H = \sum_{j=1}^{N-1} t\,[\,(f_j^{\dagger} f_{j+1}^{\dagger} + f_j^{\dagger} f_{j+1}) + (f_{j+1} f_j + f_{j+1}^{\dagger} f_j)\,]$$

$$= \sum_{j=1}^{N-1} t\,[\,f_j^{\dagger}(f_{j+1}^{\dagger} + f_{j+1}) - f_j\,(f_{j+1} + f_{j+1}^{\dagger})\,] =$$

$$\sum_{j=1}^{N-1} t\,[\,(f_j^{\dagger} - f_j)(f_{j+1} + f_{j+1}^{\dagger})\,] = -\sum_{j=1}^{N-1} t\, b_j\, a_{j+1} =$$

$$\sum_{j=1}^{N-1} t\, a_{j+1} b_j.$$

The last expression exhibits the Majorana particles belonging to the original fermions with the real part one unit ahead of the imaginary part. The resulting structure suggests defining new fermions call them $g_1, g_2, \ldots, g_{N-1}$. They are such that, $g_j = 1/2(a_{j+1} + ib_j)$, for j =1 to N-1. These new fermions are illustrated in Figure 5.1 B. In this diagram there exists two rows of smaller circles underneath the top row, They denote the real and imaginary parts of these fermions in that order. However, notice that new pairs of Majorana particles are linked together a diagonal manner to form the new Dirac fermions g_j. In this case, g_j are specified above. Also observe that in the new formulation, two Majorana particles are left out. These are the real part of f_1 to the left as well as the imaginary part of f_N to the right. Both a_1 and b_N are the MZM particles. Together, they form a new quantity $g_N = 1/2 (a_1 + ib_N)$. The MZM structure has a relatively large distance between its real and imaginary parts thereby providing topological protection.

MZM are used in quantum computing because they are naturally resistant to noise and error. They do not lose coherency as rapid as other designs. Each end holds information and together they form a qubit. Qubits are also formed using a single edge

MZM from one Kitaev chain and another one from a different Kitaev chain. Additionally, a single MZM is combined with an internal particle within the Kitaev chain, If the combined state of the two MZM is a fermion then this determines the state, zero, or one.

Again, when assuming that u = 0 and Δ = t, then the Lie product is:

$$[\,H,\ g_k\,] = [\ \sum_{j=1}^{N-1} t\, a_{j+1} b_j,\ 1/2(\, a_{k+1} + i b_k\,)\,] =$$

$$1/2 \sum_{j=1}^{N-1} (\ (\,t\, a_{j+1} b_j\, a_{k+1} + t\, a_{j+1} b_j\, i b_k\,) -$$

$$(\, a_{k+1}\, t\, a_{j+1} b_j + i b_k t\, a_{j+1} b_j)\,) = 0.$$

This follows by anti commuting Majorana particles for all indices except when j = k, or k+1, here the square of a particle is one. More generally, [H, g_k]

is proportional to e^{-rc} which is a small quantity depending on the distance between the Majoranas.

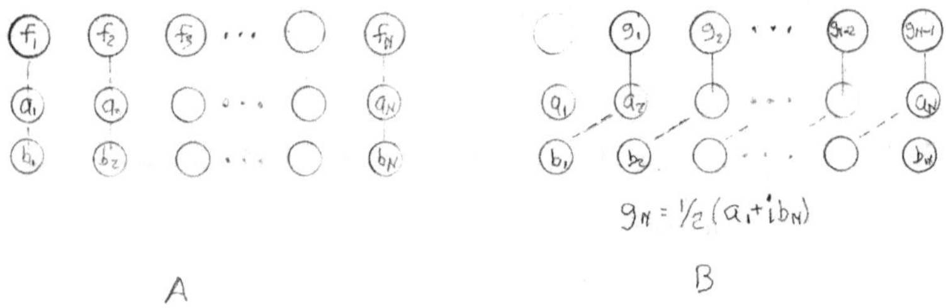

FIGURE 5.1)

5.2) Braiding Majorana Zero Modes

For two distinct Majorana Zero Mode, MZM particles, a and b there are two ways to braid them. This is best explained by fixing them in a plane and rotating them 180 degrees about a point located centrally between a and b. The rotation should be counterclockwise, and the braid will correspond to the world time path illustrated as increasing time is depicted downward. This is provided in Figure 5.2, with explanations described next.

The rotation is governed by the operator $R_{ab} = e^{(\pi/4ab)}$. (Yural, 2022). When expanded into a power series $R_{ab} = \sum_{n=0}^{\infty} 1/(n!) (\pi/4 \text{ ab})^n$. Expand this series, and utilize the identities, $a^2 = b^2 = 1$, and also ab = -ba, results in the sum of two power series, one with even terms and one with odd terms. Specifically,

$$R_{ab} = \sum_{n=0}^{\infty} (1/(2n)!) (\pi/4)^{2n} +$$

$$ab \sum_{n=0}^{\infty} (1/(2n+1)!) (\pi/4)^{(2n+1)} = \cos(\pi/4) +$$

$$ab \sin(\pi/4) = 2^{-1/2}(1 + ab).$$

Next use the defining properties of the Majorana structure, namely that $a^\dagger = a$, and $b^\dagger = b$ as well as using $(ab)^\dagger = b^\dagger a^\dagger$. Consequently, $R_{ab}^\dagger b R_{ab} = 1/2 (1 + b^\dagger a^\dagger) b (1 + ab) = 1/2 (1 - ab) b (1 + ab) = 1/2 [b - abb + bab - abbab] = 1/2 [b - a - a - b] = -a$. Similarly, $R_{ab}^\dagger a R_{ab} = b$. The actual braiding involving Majorana particles is illustrated in Figure 5.2, below. The original top plane consists of Two

Majorana particles a, and b. In the diagrams as time progresses illustrations go downward. On the left figure below f_a(a, b) = (b, -a). Note that notation provided in Section 4.1 is exclusively utilized here. Additionally, on the right, f_a^{-1}(a, b) = (b a).

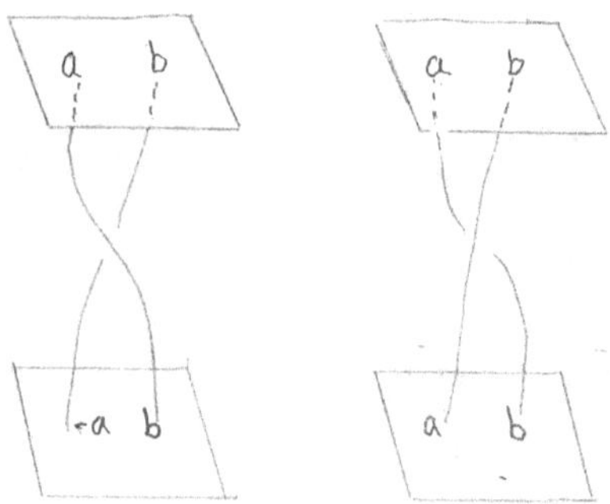

FIGURE 5.2)

Finally, notice that $R_{ab}^{\dagger}$ R_{ab} = 1/2 (1 -ab) (1 + ab) = 1. Additionally, $R_{ab}R_{ab}^{\dagger}$ = 1.

5.3) Exchanging Positions of MZMs

Recall that the Majorana particles are associated with the real and imaginary parts of a Dirac fermion. For instance, assuming that there exists four Majorana particles, a, b, c, and d. Formally, two different fermions using a pair of Majorana particles only once, can be constructed in 120 distinct ways. This is because, using four Majorana particles there are twelve ways a single pair of Majorana particles can be constructed. Here no two particles constitute the same Dirac fermion. Any of the four particles can represent either the real part, or the imaginary part. The second structure cannot utilize both particles existing in the first fermion. However it can use one of them in the real or imaginary location. There are ten ways this can happen, resulting in 120 possibilities. Figure 5.3, illustrates four Majorana particles located as corners of a square. Rigorously, they can be grouped as couples in six ways, however the end points of these groupings can be in the real part or the imaginary part of a Dirac fermion. Once a first fermion is chosen, there are only five groupings remaining. See Figure 5.3 . For instance, a + bi can be the first Dirac fermion, and the second could be c + ai. (Ivanov, 2001).

FIGURE 5.3)

Suppose that the first fermion is f_{ab} = 1/2(a + ib), and the second is f_{cd} = 1/2 (c +id). In this case, a = f_{ab} + $f_{ab}^{\dagger}$, b = i($f_{ab}^{\dagger}$ - f_{ab}), moreover, $a^{\dagger}$ = $f_{ab}^{\dagger}$ + $f_{ab}^{\dagger\dagger}$ = a. Similarly, $b^{\dagger}$ = -i($f_{ab}^{\dagger\dagger}$ - $f_{ab}^{\dagger}$) = b. Additionally, c = f_{cd} + $f_{cd}^{\dagger}$, and d = i($f_{cd}^{\dagger}$ - f_{cd}). The objective now is to exchange Majorana particles b and c. To do this use R_{bc}, and by analogy from the last section, $R_{bc}^{\dagger}$b R_{bc}= c, also $R_{bc}^{\dagger}$c R_{bc} = -b. Since there are two distinct fermions each can be in a single configuration with an occupied state or empty state. The two fermions can have either even or odd parity state situations.

The even parity states are $| 0_{ab}, \; 0_{cd} >$, and $| 1_{ab}, 1_{cd} >$. The first configuration is the empty state, and the second is where both positions have a single fermion, In a similar manner the odd parity states are where only a single position is occupied, thus, $| 1_{ab}, \; 0_{cd} >$, and $| 0_{ab}, \; 1_{cd} >$ are odd.

Recall that an annihilation operator for instance, f_{ab} operating on the empty state results in zero, that is $f_{ab} [0_{ab} > = 0$. Also the creation operation $f_{ab}^{\dagger}$ is such that $f_{ab}^{\dagger} \; | \; 0_{ab} > = | \; 1_{ab} >$. Exchange the location of MZM b, and c at the state $| \; 0_{ab}, \; 0_{cd} >$. Formally, the operation needed is $R_{bc}^{\dagger} | \; 0_{ab}, \; 0_{cd} >$. Using the operator $R_{bc}^{\dagger} = \; 2^{-1/2} [\, 1 - bc \,] \, | \, 0_{ab}, \; 0_{cd} > \; = \; 2^{-1/2} [\, 1 - i(\; f_{ab}^{\dagger} - \; f_{ab})(\, f_{cd} + f_{cd}^{\dagger}) \,] \, | \, 0_{ab}, \; 0_{cd} > \; = \; 2^{-1/2} [\, 1 - i(\; f_{ab}^{\dagger} f_{cd} \; + \; f_{ab}^{\dagger} f_{cd}^{\dagger} - f_{ab} f_{cd} - f_{ab} f_{cd}^{\dagger} \,) \,] \, | \, 0_{ab}, \; 0_{cd} > = 2^{-1/2} [\, 1 - i(\; f_{ab}^{\dagger} f_{cd}^{\dagger} \,)] | \, 0_{ab}, \; 0_{cd} > = 2^{-1/2} [\, | \, 0_{ab}, \; 0_{cd} > -i \, | \, 1_{ab}, \; 1_{cd} >]$. This state is located on the equator on the Bloch sphere, and is illustrated in Figure 5.4. In this diagram the North Pole is denoted by $| \; 0_{ab}, \; 0_{cd} >$, while the South Pole is described by $| \, 1_{ab}, \; 1_{cd} >$. Only six states can be developed by the above procedure.

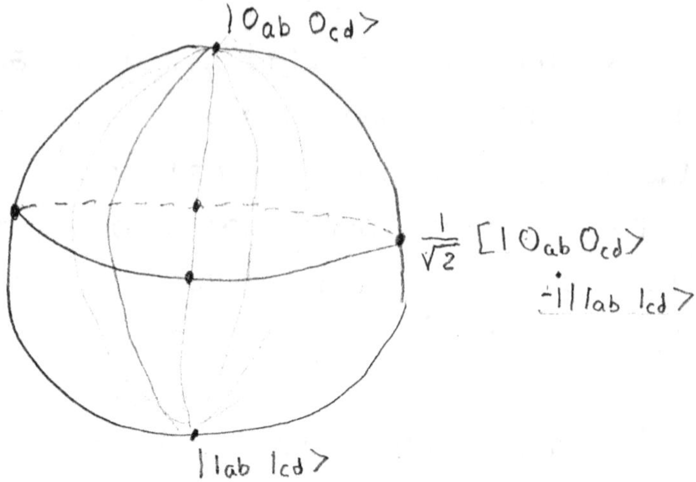

FIGURE 5.4)

Majorana quasiparticles have topological properties and are proposed as being a collection of fermions in a cooled down material. The collective behavior of bunches of fermions act like their own anti particle. This provides a topological protection. In a superconductor Cooper Pairs arise, they are pairs of fermions. The braiding of particles holds the information. Majorana particles are often mistaken to be Cooper pairs. Cooper pairs have zero sum spin and have mass and charge twice that of a single electron. The momentum in each electron within a Cooper pair is equal and opposite in sign. They have power energy less than the Fermi energy, and as such thermal energy can break the bonding. Large groupings of Cooper pairs are therefore, found at low temperatures. Accordingly, the pair is said to be bound in conventional super-conductance caused by electron photon interaction. The quantum effect creates super conducting. This bunching or pairing, but the binding is weak. Accordingly, only at low temperatures are there numerous BCS pairs

In (Maciazek and Conlon, 2023) deep learning techniques are used in finding optimal control protocols for exchanging MZM in realizing topological quantum computers. Exchanges are performed on networks consisting of coupled p wave superconducting nanowires. Fine tuning of gradient techniques in neural networks are employed in the optimization strategy.

APPENDIX 1) FOCK SPACES

A1.1 Fock Spaces for Bosons and Fermions

Fock space is a direct sum of tensor products of Hilbert spaces. It is used in representing various states of identical particle Hilbert spaces H. All eements are indistinguishable from one another in a fixed Fock space. The major type of particles described in Fock spaces are bosons and fermions. Other particles such as negatively charged ions, like anyonic particles are not described in this space. For bosons a sum of symmetrized tensor product of n single particle Hilbert spaces are employed. Zero particle states, single particle states, two particle states, … . These all are a tensor product of H with itself. The quantity $(\otimes \text{ H })^n$, is the tensor product of H, n times. In short, Fock space F will be written in this section in the following manner, it is, F = (+) [S $(\otimes \text{ H })^n$]. Here, n = 0, 1, 2, …, and the operator (+) stands for the direct sum from 0 to infinity. So, expanding the above expression in more detail, gives, F = C + H + S (H ⊗ H) + S (H ⊗ H ⊗ H) + … . In this representation the plus, + , is used for

the direct sum of two individual terms. The quantity C, is the field of complex numbers denoting the vacuum state, and it is abbreviated, vac. Vac is the state consisting of no particles.
For bosonic Fock space S is symmetry operation, for fermionic it is antisymmetric. The Hilbert space, H is the state for single particles, while S (H ⊗ H) describes the states for two identical particles. The two identical particle state is also denoted by S H2. Similarly, S (H ⊗ H ⊗ H) describes the states for three identical particles, and it will be denoted by S H3, and so on.

Finally, identify a vector v in Hj by the jth tuple of (0, 0, ..., 0, v, 0, ...), and use the notation v = vj. Also, the space Hj is orthogonal to the space Hi whenever j does not equal the integer value i. The latter statement means that the n particle subspaces for different values of n are orthogonal.

It is useful to provide an additional, but related concept of a state for Fock space. Begin with the symmetric Fock space, it must always be infinite dimensional. For a finite dimensional Hilbert space

H1, consider an observable having eigenvectors I ej >, j = 1, 2, … , n, and corresponding eigenvalues aj. When a single particle occupies the kth state this means that the eigenstate ket, I ek > = I 0, 0, …, 0, 1, 0, … 0 >, and where the one appears in the kth position. Correspondingly, with similar assumptions the two particle space H2, could have both particles in a single state, or a single particle in two distinct states among the n states. So, for instance in bosonic Fock space, the possibilities for two particles in a single state are: both in the first state, I 2, 0, …, 0 >, or both in the second state, I 0, 2, 0, …, 0 >, and so on to the last state I 0, …, 0, 2 >. Additionally, in any Fock space the two particles can be separated: I 1, 1, 0 …, 0 >, I 1, 0, 1, 0, …, 0 >, …, I 0, … 0, 1, 1 >. Theses are all the possible state occupancies for two particles. An important thing to realize is that H2 is not the tensor product of H1, and H1. It is isomorphic to the symmetrized direct sum of tensor products, that is: H = S (H1⊗ H1). Briefly, in this case S (ha ⊗ hb) = (ha ⊗ hb) + (hb ⊗ ha). Similarly, in H3 there would be a direct sum of three factorial tensored products, that is six possibilities. Linear combinations of product states is the general state in Fock space.

Example A1.1)
Consider H2, this is a two particle Hilbert space, using distinct kets { I 0 >, I 0' > }. As seen previously there exists four possible states involving these two kets, these distinct states are given by: { I 0 0 >, I 0 0' >, I 0' 0' >, I 0' 0 > }. Each state has equal probability of being assembled, but not observed. There exist three symmetrical states for observation and a single anti symmetrical state. These are in order, I 0 0 >, I 0' 0' >, I 0 0' > + I 0' 0 >, and I 0 0' > - I 0' 0 >. The first three are bosonic states, they are similar to the form, S (ha ⊗ hb) = (ha ⊗ hb) + (hb ⊗ ha). The last expression will be shown to be a fermionic state.#

A1.2 Bosonic Creation and Annihilation

In Fock space there exists transitions between particles within sub spaces of distinct number. Thus particle numbers are not preserved, particles can be created or destroyed, that is annihilated. These elements can be added or removed from any given energy state. Operators corresponding to these functions are called ladder operations. In quantum mechanics, these transitions caused by the ladder operators are referred to as second quantization, and involve the blending of Hilbert subspaces Hn and H(n+-1). The operators have arguments which are particles like photons or quasiparticles like phonons. The foundation of bosonic Fock space is the Bose-Einstein statistics.

The bosonic Fock space algebra over the Hilbert space H allows all states to be occupied by n, where n is any finite number of particles. That is n = 0, 1, ... In this space, the number operator Nj, provides the count of the number of particles for the jth eigenstate. This operator keeps track of the quantity of particles that are located in every state. The occupational number nj, for an observable A, along with non negative integer valued eigenvalues is such that Nj (I n0, n1, n2, ..., nj,..., nk >) = nj I n0, n1, ..., nj, ..., nk >. Accordingly, for the operator, Nj, the eigenvector is In0, n1, n2, ..., nj,..., nk >, and the corresponding eigenvalue is the occupational number, nj. The observable A, can be written as a sum, $\sum_{j}$ (cj Nj), where the cj are scalars.

The creation operation is employed in Fock space to add a particle in the prescribed quantum state, j. This operator is denoted by $aj^{\dagger}$, it focuses on the jth state only, and increments the occupancy number of this state by one. This operation on the quantum state is an exterior or symmetric multiplication. Specifically, $aj^{\dagger}$ (I ..., nj, ... >) = (nj + 1 $)^{1/2}$ (I ..., nj + 1, ... >). The parenthesis will often be left out for these operators in the following. Opposite to the creation operator is the annihilator operator aj.

In general, the creation operator adds a particle whenever a particle is present or not. For a non vacant state the annihilation operation will decrement the occupation number by one. However, when the jth state is empty the annihilation operator performed on this state will result with zero. When the annihilator acts on the vacuum state C, that is vac, the result will also be zero. In summary, for non vacant states, aj I ..., nj,

...> = $nj^{1/2}$ I ..., nj - 1, ...,>, when nj is positive, and this yields zero otherwise.

There are numerous relationships between the creation operator, $a^\dagger$, the annihilation operator, a, and the number N, operator. Before these relations are identified it will be assumed that the creation operation and the annihilation operations are adjoints of one another. That is $a^\dagger = a^*$, and $(a^\dagger)^* = a$. These facts are justified in the C* algebra of the Banach space completion for the bosonic Fock space. (Townsend, 2000). Now use the non vacuum and occupied state with n particles. Here, $a^\dagger a$ I n > = $n^{1/2} a^\dagger$I n-1 > = $n^{1/2}$ $n^{1/2}$ I n > = N I n >. Thus the identification between the number operator and both the creation and annihilation operations is $N = a^\dagger a$. In a similar fashion, $a\, a^\dagger$ I n > = $(n+1)^{1/2}$ a I n + 1 > = $(n+1)^{1/2}(n+1)^{1/2}$ I n > = (n +1) I n >. It follows that $a\, a^\dagger$ acts like (N + I). This is the number operator plus the identity map. Commutation relations are a consequence of the identities just given. The commutator, $[a, a^\dagger] = a\, a^\dagger - a^\dagger a = (N + I) - N = I$. Additionally, $[N, a^\dagger] = N a^\dagger - a^\dagger N = a^\dagger a\, a^\dagger - a^\dagger a^\dagger a = a^\dagger (a\, a^\dagger - a^\dagger a) =$

$a^\dagger$ (I) = $a^\dagger$. Similarly, [N, a] = N a - a N = $a^\dagger$ a a - a $a^\dagger$ a = ($a^\dagger$ a - a $a^\dagger$) a = - a.

Example A1.2)

The ground state of zero can be algebraically explained using the ladder operators using the fact that the operators a, and $a^\dagger$ are mutually adjoint. Here, for the annihilation operation energy eigenstates can only be lowered to zero, and never less than this amount. To see that the minimum eigen number is zero, consider N = $a^\dagger$ a, and N ϕ_n = n ϕ_n. Then < ϕ_n I N ϕ_n > = < ϕ_n I $a^\dagger$ a ϕ_n > = < a ϕ_n I a ϕ_n > = , II a I ϕ_n > II^2, which is non negative and equals zero iff a I ϕ_n > = 0, and so for n = 0, again, it shown that, a I ϕ_0 > = 0.#

Basic Fock states with n bosons are given by the cyclic property of the creation operation: ($a^\dagger$)^n I 0 >, where n is a positive integer. These Fock states usually do not contain any information as to the phase. However, the bosonic coherent state v, is in essence a Gaussian wave packet. It is a special bosonic state, and involves the annihilation operator a. Specifically it is the eigenstate of a. So, a v = r v, where r is the eigenvalue and since v is a state, it is assumed that $\| v \| = 1$. Coherent states have dynamics similar to classical oscillatory trajectories and are related to the quantum harmonic oscillations. (Gazeau, 2009)

A1.3 Fermionic Creation and Annihilation

The occupation number in the case of fermionic Fock space is trivial because N can only be zero or one. The foundation of fermionic Fock space are the Pauli exclusion principal and the Fermi-Dirac statistics. In this case, either there exists a particle in a given state or there is none. The occupation operator is a binary function in the fermionic Fock space. The ladder operators $a^\dagger$, and a, in the fermionic Fock space are similar to those in the bosonic Fock space. Intuitively, as before the creation operator $a^\dagger$, adds a particle to a state, but in this space the state has to be empty. The annihilation operator removes a particle from a state, provided there is a single particle to be annihilated. The anti communication relations providing the fermionic Fock space algebra is given by the Poisson bracket: { ai, aj } = ai aj + aj ai = 0, for all states i and j, also { $ai^\dagger$, $aj^\dagger$ } = 0, and finally, { ai, $aj^\dagger$ } = 0, except that it equals one when i = j. As a consequence of the first two identities it follows that a a = $a^\dagger$ $a^\dagger$ = 0. The number operator as in the bosonic case is given by N = $a^\dagger a$. However, since { a $a^\dagger$ + $a^\dagger$ a } = 1, then a $a^\dagger$ = 1 - N. From this, N (1 - N) = $a^\dagger$ a a $a^\dagger$ = 0. So the eigenvalues for N are either zero or one. This confirms the Pauli principle that the occupation number is zero or one. It can be seen that the eigenstates of N are $a^\dagger$ | 0 >, and a | 1 > with corresponding eigenvalues 1 and 0 respectively. These results follow since (1 - N) $a^\dagger$ | 0 > = a $a^\dagger$ $a^\dagger$ | 0 > = 0, as well as N a | 1 > = $a^\dagger$ a a | 1 > = 0.

In two dimensional Hilbert space with orthonormal basis { | 0 >, | 1 > }. It follows that a | 0 > = $a^\dagger$ | 1 > = 0, $a^\dagger$ | 0 > = | 1 >, finally, a | 1 > = | 0 >. Note that a = | 0 >< 1 |, because a | 0 > = | 0 >< 1 | 0 > = 0, also a | 1 > = | 0 >< 1 | 1 > = | 0 >. Correspondingly, for the creation operation $a^\dagger$ = | 1 >< 0 |, since, $a^\dagger$ |1 > = | 1 >< 0 | 1 > = 0, and $a^\dagger$ | 0 > = | 1 >< 0 | 0 > = |

$1\rangle$. Also, $a\, a = |0\rangle\langle 1|0\rangle\langle 1| = 0$, and $a^\dagger a^\dagger = |1\rangle\langle 0|1\rangle\langle 0| = 0$. As a consequence,, neither a nor $a^\dagger$ are self adjoint, however they are conjugate adjoint. That is, $(a)^* = a^\dagger$, because $(|0\rangle\langle 1|)^* = |1\rangle\langle 0|$, similarly, $(a^\dagger)^* = a$.

In the Hilbert space C^2, it was seen that the representations for $|0\rangle$, and $|1\rangle$ are given by the column vectors (1 0)' and (0 1)' respectively. In this space two by two matrices for the creation operation $a^\dagger$, and annihilation operation a, are given in order by:

$$\begin{vmatrix} 0 & 0 \\ 1 & 0 \end{vmatrix} \qquad \begin{vmatrix} 0 & 1 \\ 0 & 0 \end{vmatrix}.$$

Using these matrices and the column vectors above, again it is seen that $a^\dagger |0\rangle = (0 \;\; 1)' = |1\rangle$, and, $a^\dagger |1\rangle = 0$, $a |0\rangle = 0$, and $a |1\rangle = (1 \;\; 0)' = |0\rangle$.

In a fermionic Hilbert space with n states there is 2^n dimensions. Moreover, each transposition of elements results in an overall negation. This follows due to the anti commutation of creation operations a †j and a†k. That is exchanging j and k creates an opposite sign, from + to - or conversely. For instance, I nj, nk > = $aj^\dagger ak^\dagger$ I vac > = - I nk, nj >. Here vac is the vacuum state.

Example A1.3)
In H3, this is a Fermionic Fock space with 3 distinct allowable states. The Hilbert space consisting of potentially of three identical fermions. So, I nj, nk, nm > spans the space. In this case the distinct possibilities are eight in number. They are I 0, 0, 0 >, I 0, 0, 1 >, I 0, 1, 0 >, I 1, 0, 0 >, I 0, 1, 1 >, I 1, 1, 0 >, I 1, 0, 1 >, I 1, 1, 1 >. Also since I nj, nk, nm > = $aj^\dagger ak^\dagger am^\dagger$ I vac >, then $ak^\dagger aj^\dagger$ $am^\dagger$I vac > = - $aj^\dagger$ ak*$am^\dagger$ I vac >. However, notice that l$ak^\dagger am^\dagger aj^\dagger$I vac > = $aj^\dagger ak^\dagger am^\dagger$I vac >, since there are two transpositions. In this case the sign changes twice.#

For a general fermionic Fock state I f > = I n1, ,n2, …, nj, …, nk, … >, the creation operation is such that $aj^\dagger$ I f > = I n1, n2, …, nj + 1, …> when nj = 0, and the result is zero otherwise. The annihilation operation using $| f \rangle$ above, is such that $aj\, | f \rangle = | n1, n2, \ldots, nj - 1, \ldots \rangle$ this occurs only when $nj = 1$, and the result is zero otherwise. To move a particles position from the jth location to an empty location say k, then an annihilation must be performed on the particle in the jth position and a creation of a particle on the kth position. In this strict order, and do not forget all particles here are identical. So, $ak^{\dagger} aj\, | f \rangle = | n1, n2, \ldots, nj -1, \ldots nk +1, \ldots \rangle = | g \rangle$. Note that $aj\, ak^{\dagger} | f \rangle = - ak^{\dagger} aj\, | f \rangle = - | g \rangle$. The identity operator in fermionic Fock space is I = product for $k = 1, 2, ..$ of $\{ ak, ak^{\dagger} \}$.

Example A1.4)
In fermionic Fock space H2 the resolution of the identity is given by $I = \{ a, a^{\dagger} \} = a\, a^{\dagger} + a^{\dagger} a = | 0 \rangle\langle 1 | 1 \rangle\langle 0 | + | 1 \rangle\langle 0 | 0 \rangle\langle 1 | = | 0 \rangle\langle 0 | + | 1 \rangle\langle 1 |$. Notice that $a\, a^{\dagger} I = a | 1 \rangle\langle 0 | (| 0 \rangle\langle 0 | + | 1 \rangle\langle 1 |) = a | 1 \rangle\langle 0 | = | 0 \rangle\langle 1 | 1 \rangle\langle 0 | = | 0 \rangle\langle 0 |$, this is a projection onto the first component of I. Also, $a^{\dagger} a\, I = a^{\dagger} | 0 \rangle\langle 1 | (| 0 \rangle\langle 0 | + | 1 \rangle\langle 1 |) = a^{\dagger} | 0 \rangle\langle 1 | = | 1 \rangle\langle 0 | 0 \rangle\langle 1 | = | 1 \rangle\langle 1 |$, this is a projection onto the second component of I.#

Consider C^2, but this time let | 0 > = (1   0)' denote the vacuum state. And let |1 > = (0   1)' represent the occupied state in this Fock space. The number operator n, along again with the creation operator $a^\dagger$ and the annihilator operation a, are all illustrated as the 2 by 2 matrices provided in order below:

| 0   0 | | 0   0 |
| 0   1 |
| 0   1 | | 1   0 |
| 0   0 |.

Note that $a^\dagger a$ = n, by multiplying the second matrix above by the third to yield the first matrix. The Poisson bracket operator gives { a, $a^\dagger$ } = $aa^\dagger + a^\dagger a$ = I. As well as $a^\dagger$| 0 > = | 1 >, $a^\dagger$ | 1 > 0, a | 0 >= 0, and finally a | 1 > = | 0 >.

APPENDIX 2 HOMOTOPY AND FUNDAMENTAL GROUPS

In a path connected topological manifold X, any two points within X can be connected by a continuous curve. More importantly, a loop consists of a continuous curve which starts at any given point and ends at that same point. Specifically, for any point p in X there is a continuous function $f_{p,q'}$: [0, 1] —-> X such that, $f_{p,q}(0) = f_{p,q}(1) = p$. Here, the q subscript implies there can be any number of continuous functions creating the loop. Note that the point itself is a loop, $f_{p,q}(t) = p$ tor all t in [0, 1], $f_{p,q}(t)$ is the constant function. Two loops $f_{p,q'}$ and $f_{p,q'}$, are homotopically equal means that the curve formed by $f_{p,q}$ can continuously be converted into the curve formed by $f_{p,q'}$. A rigorous treatment of Homotopic and group concepts is provided in (Giardina, 2024).

Example 2.1)

In the Euclidean x-y plane, R^2 for any point p all loops are homotopic to each other. These curves are said to be equivalent.#

Example 2.2)
On the unit circle S^1, in the Euclidean x-y plane, not all loops are homotopic to each other. For instance, the first curve $f_{p,q}$ starts at p = (1, 0). It goes counterclockwise staying on the circle to the top point (0, 1) and returns clockwise to point p. It is not homotopic to the different curve $f_{p,q'}$ which starts at p and goes a full 360 degrees counterclockwise back to p.#

The fundamental group of a topological connected manifold is comprised of all the distinct equivalence classes within the structure. An equivalence class consists of all loops which can be continuously deformed into each other.

Example 2.3)
The fundamental group for S^1 given in Example 2.2, is equivalent to the group of all integers Z, with the usual addition law. In this case, an integer n is

assigned to the winding number. That is, the number of times a path goes full revolution around the circle counterclockwise starting and ending at point p. Clockwise revolutions are specified by negative integers. Finally, the integer 0 represents loops which never go around the circle a full 360 degrees.#

Example 2.4)

A torus, or donut is illustrated in Figure A2.1. On this diagram are illustrations of three loops. Loop 1 denotes any loop which does not go a full circle enclosing the torus. It lies on the left top in this case. Loop 2 represents any loop in the vertical type position, like slicing a donut. Loop 3 indicates a somewhat larger loop going around the entire donut slicing it in a somewhat horizontal manner. The set of all loops within the torus first appears to be a free group. To see this let v denote any vertical loop similar to loop 2, and let h represent any horizontal loop corresponding to the loop 3. Additionally let $v^0 = h^0 = I$, standing for the identity mapping and representing any loop equivalent to Loop 1.

For any integers p and q assume that v^p means that p full revolution wraparounds in the vertical occur in the direction indicated. For negative p the opposite direction is assumed. Similarly q horizontal loops occurs using h^q. For instance in the diagram to the right of v, v^{-2} is illustrated. So for instance the word: $Iv^{-3}h^2v^4hv^2h$, reading right to left, means that a single horizontal loop is followed by two vertical loops. This is followed by a horizontal loop and then by four vertical loops and then by two horizontal loops. Finally three opposite direction vertical loops are followed by the identity loop I. The free group consists of all such words. However, notice that any vertical loop must intersect a horizontal loop at some point on the torus. A consequence is that it doesn't matter if the vertical occurs first followed by a horizontal loop or the other way around. Thus the group is commutative, that is vh = hv. Various powers of v and h also commute.

Since the group is Abelian the expression $Iv^{-3}h^2v^4$ hv^2h can be simplified, it can be written: $v^{-3}v^4v^2h^2h$ $h = v^3h^4$. The last expression can be represented as the pair of integers (3, 4). Thus this group is equivalent to Z x Z, the set of two tuples of integers.#

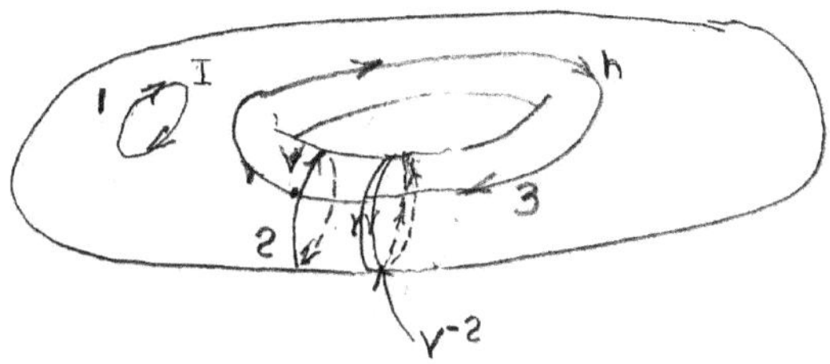

FIGURE A2.1

REFERENCES

Alicia, J., et al Non-Abelian statistics and topological quantum information, Nature Physics, 2011.

Alicia, J., New directions in the pursuit of Majorana fermions in solid state systems ArXiv, 2024.

All Nobel Prizes, The Nobel Prize, 2024.

Amaldi, E., From the discovery of the neutron to the discovery of nuclear fission, Physics Reports 1984.

Apple, S., Ravenous: Otto Warburg, the Nazis and the search for the cancer-diet connection, 2021.

Biswas, S., Fermi Dirac Statistics, arXiv, 2015.

Bose, S., Planck's law and the hypothesis of light quanta, Dacca, U, India, 1924.

Castelvecchi, D., Microsoft claims quantum-computing breakthrough—but physicists are skeptical, Nature 2025.

Chenn, I., and Sigal, I., The Bogolubov de Gennes, equations of superconductivity, ArXiv, 2019.

Connover, E., Physicists are mostly unconvinced by Microsoft's new topological chip. ScienceNews, 2025.

Duraj, T., et al, Clinical research framework proposal for ketogenic metabolic therapy in glioblastoma, BMC Medicine 2024.

Fox, J., ' This is essentially a fraudulent project' Some scientists are firing shots at Microsoft's recent computing claims. PCGamer, 2025.

Frolic, Quantum Transport Lecture 12 Spin Qubits (Frolov, 2014)

Fu, I., and Kane, C., Superconducting proximity effect and Majorana Fermions at the surface of a topological insulator, PRL, 100, 2008.

Garisto, D., Controversial quantum-computing paper gets hefty correction-but concerns linger, Nature, 2025.

Garisto, D., Microsoft quantum computing 'breakthrough' faces fresh challenge, Nature, 2025.

Gazeau, J., Coherent states in quantum physics, Wiley, 2009.

Giardina, C., Many-Sorted Algebras for Deep Learning and Quantum Technology. Elsevier, 2024.

Giardina, C., Probability for Deep Learning Quantum, A Many-Sorted Algebra View, Elsevier, 2025.

Giardina, C., AI Cancer Timebomb, Regency Publishing Co. 2025.

Giardina, C., Mysteries of the Mitochondria, Regency Publishing Co. 2025.

Giardina, C., Theronostics, Regency Publishing Co. 2025.

Helmenstine, A., Pauli Exclusion Principle, Science Notes and Projects, 2022.

Jainendra, J., Q&A: Will Microsoft's quantum 'breakthrough' revolutionize computing? PennState, 2025.

Ivanov, D. Non-Abelian statistics of half-quantum vortices in p-wave superconductors, Phys Rev Lett, 2001.

Kiessaling, M., Do particles and antiparticles really annihilate each other? U Texas, Austin, 2018.

Lee, D, et al, Amino acid and glucose fermentation maintain ATP content in mouse and human malignant glioma cells, Nearo, 2024.

Lee, S., The physics behind excitons: a deep dive, Number Analytics, 2025.

Li, Y., et al, Invasion and metastasis in cancer molecular insights and therapeutic targets, Signal Transduction and Targeted Therapy, 2025.

LibreTexts, The properties of protons, neutrons and electrons, 2019.

LibreTexts, Negative Energies and antiparticles, 2025

Maciazek, T., and Conlon, M., Optimizing the exchange of Majorana zero modes in a quantum nanowire network, ArXiv, 2023.

Madison, K., et al, Vortex formation in a stirred Bose-Einstein condensate, APS2000

Mann, A., Corrected study rekindles debate over Microsofts's quantum computing research, Science, 2025.

Monti, N., et al, Paradoxical behavior of oncogenes undermines the somatic mutation theory, NIH, 2022.

Mourik, V.,et al, Signatures of Majorana fermions in hybrid superconductor- superconductor nanowire devices, 2012.

Yural, O., Braiding Majorana Zero Modes, Whzmann Institute of Science, 2022.

Pasayten.org, Up and down quarks, 2025

Recami, E., Majorana, the neutron, and the neutrino: some elementary historical remarks, Semantic Scholar, 2017.

Reid, S., Examples of fundamental groups, StackExchange, Mathematics, 2014.

Rouabah, M., Compiling single-qubit braiding gate for Fibonacci anyons topological quantum computation, ArXiv, 2008.

Rouabah, M., et al, Compiling single-qubit braiding gate for Fibonacci anyons topological quantum computation, J of Physics, 2020.

Ruelle, M., et al, Time-domain braiding of anyons, ArXiv, 2024.

Scienceinfo.net, Ettore Majorana-The genius physicist who disappeared mysteriously, 2025.

Seyfried, T., and Shelton, L., Cancer as a metabolic disease. Nutr Metab, London, 2010.

Seyfried, T., et al, Metabolic management of brain cancer, Elsevier, 2011.

Seyfried, T, et al Cancer as a metabolic disease: implications for novel therapeutics, Carcinogenesis, Vol 35 no 3, 2014.

Seyfried, T., Cancer as a mitochondrial metabolic disease, Frontiers in Cell and Developmental Biology, 2015.

Seyfried, T., et al, Metabolic therapy: a new paradigm for managing malignant brain cancer, Cancer Lett 2015

Seyfried, T., et al Considerations of ketogenic metabolic therapy as a complementary or alternative approach for managing breast cancer, Frontiers in Nutrition, 2020.

Seyfried, T., Ketogenic metabolic therapy, without chemo or radiation, NIH, 2021.

Seyfried, T., et al, On the origin go ATP synthesis in cancer, iScience, 2022.

Seyfried, T., et al, The Warburg hypothesis and the emergence of the mitochondrial metabolic theory of cancer, JBB 2025.

Shelton, L., et al, Glutamine targeting inhibits systematic metastasis in the VM-M3 murine tumor model, NIH, 2010.

The Nobel Prize Internet Archive,W hy is there no Nobel Prize in Mathematics? 1996.

Townsend, J., A modern approach to quantum mechanics,

University Science Books, 2000

U of Rhode Island, Fermion operators and hopping bands, Phys.uni.edu, 2011.

Weber, G., Metabolism in cancer metastasis, NIH, 2016.

ABOUT THE AUTHOR

Dr. Giardina was a professor of mathematics, electrical engineering, and computer science at Fairleigh Dickinson University from 1965 to 1982. From 1982 to 1986, he was a professor at the Stevens Institute of Technology. On behalf of these two universities he headed off campus programs at various industrial and military locations, such as Fort Monmouth, ITT, Bendix, Bell Labs, Bellcore, and Kearfott, all in NJ.From 1986 to 1999, he was a professor at the College of Staten Island, City University of New York.

His industrial career began at Transil Semiconductors, Englewood NJ in 1963. Subsequently he was awarded a Communication Development Training fellowship at Bell Telephone Laboratories, Whippany, NJ, United States where he worked in military defense. He continued in the area of military defense and research in 1968 at Singer Kearfott, Wayne NJ. Later in 1996, he again joined Bell Telephone Laboratories, Whippany, NJ, United States. Finally, in 1998, Dr. Giardina returned to Kearfott, then called BAE Systems as a Senior Member of the Technical Staff.

His research interests include digital signal and image processing, pattern recognition, artificial intelligence, and the constructive theory of functions. Dr. Giardina has authored numerous papers and several books in these areas, including Mathematical Models for Artificial Intelligence and Autonomous Systems, Prentice Hall; Matrix Structure Image Processing, Prentice Hall; Parallel Digital Signal Processing: A Unified Signal Algebra Approach, Regency; Morphological Methods in Image and Signal Processing, Prentice Hall; Image Processing—Continuous to Discrete: Geometric, Transform, and Statistical Methods, Prentice Hall; and A Unified Signal Algebra Approach to Two-Dimensional Parallel Digital Signal Processing, Chapman and Hall/CRC Press. Most recently he authored: Many-Sorted Algebras for Deep Learning and Quantum Technology, Feb 2024, Elsevier; Probability for Deep Learning Quantum, A Many-Sorted Algebra View, Jan 2025, Elsevier; AI Cancer Timebomb, Regency, May 2025. Mysteries of the

Mitochondria, Regency, July 2025. Theranostics, Regency, August 2025.

DEDICATION

To Betty, My Everything.

ACKNOWLEDGMENTS

Thanks goes to Ed Cooke for reading the manuscript and making excellent corrections, as well as valuable suggestions.

Thanks also to Brian Moseley, from the Apple Store in San Luis Obispo. Without his help, page numbers would not exist.

A very special thank you to Manouri Nissanka for an ingenious reconfiguration of the front cover.